Calm Your Inflammation-Anti-Inflammatory Diet

A Science-Backed Plan to Enhance Your Immune System, Promote Gut Health, Boost Energy, and Feel Your Best Every Day

Dr. Brenda Tidwell

The information in this book is intended to be educational and not for diagnosis, prescription, or treatment of any health disorder. The advice and strategies contained herein may not be suitable for your situation. This information should not replace consultation with a competent healthcare professional. The content of this publication is intended to be used as an adjunct to a rational and responsible healthcare program prescribed by a healthcare practitioner. All effort has been executed to present accurate, up to date, complete, and reliable information. No warranties of any kind are declared or implied. The author is in no way liable for any misuse of the material.

1st edition 2024

To my husband,

Your unwavering love, support, and encouragement have been my foundation and inspiration throughout our many years of marriage.

Thank you for being my greatest champion, my trusted advisor, and my constant reminder of what truly matters.

I love you.

A Gift to My Readers

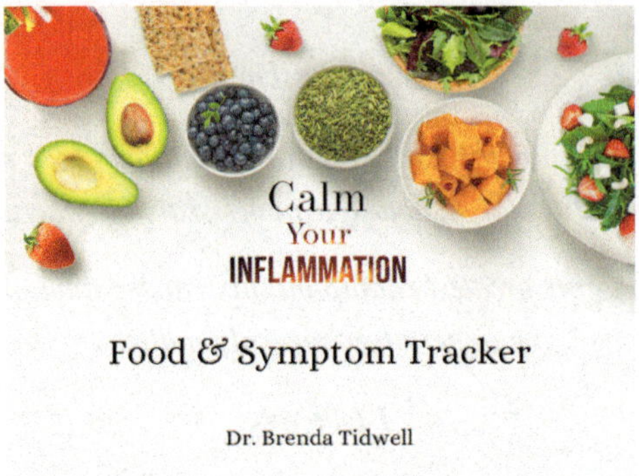

Take the first step toward a healthier, inflammation-free life! Download our exclusive Food and Symptom Tracker, a perfect companion for the Calm Your Inflammation series. My easy-to-use tracker will help you identify the foods that trigger your symptoms and discover a way of eating that works for you. Follow this link or scan the QR code to get your free tracker and begin transforming your health!

https://fireside-publications.kit.com/fb73dd7e03

To get your free downloadable Food and Symptom Tracker, you can follow the URL, or just scan this QR code with the camera on your phone and touch the link that pops up. The rest is even easier! Just follow the prompts.

Contents

Introduction

In today's fast-paced world, where fast-food restaurants outnumber farmers' markets, it's no wonder chronic inflammation affects so many people. This health epidemic, linked with a myriad of chronic diseases, can undermine our health and happiness. Yet, amidst this prevalent concern lies a pathway to calm your inflammation—a transformative journey that begins at the end of your fork.

As a Doctor of Nursing Practice and a board-certified Family Nurse Practitioner, I am deeply committed to wellness and healing. I have devoted my career and personal life to unraveling the complexities of chronic disease and discovering practical, life-changing solutions for those in my care. I am deeply passionate about educating others on combating inflammation and enhancing overall health and well-being.

I wrote this book as a practical guide to help simplify complex dietary changes. It complements my previous work, "Calm Your Inflammation." Together, these books offer hope and actionable strategies for those suffering from inflammation-linked chronic diseases and those who wish to avoid chronic inflammation and its potentially devastating effects. This guide is designed with the beginner in mind, offering stress-free meal planning and adaptable recipes to suit various dietary needs—all backed by scientific insights to validate the effectiveness of this approach.

I understand the hurdles that come with dietary changes, especially when managing inflammation. Perhaps you've tried changing your diet before but felt overwhelmed by complex recipes or the extensive prep work involved. Or maybe you're concerned about the cost and time. This book was designed to ease those concerns and guide you through each step.

Allow me to share a quick story. One of my patients struggled with rheumatoid arthritis, which made even the simplest tasks unbearably painful. After adopting an anti-inflammatory way of eating, she experienced a reduction in her symptoms. She was able to enjoy eating and preparing food that contributed to her health and resulted in fewer painful days. Her story is a reminder of the transformative nature of the foods we choose to eat.

As we move forward, remember that this book is not just about eliminating certain foods from your plate; it's about discovering a world of foods and flavors that can heal, nourish, and rejuvenate your body. By the end, you'll have the tools to prepare easy, delicious anti-inflammatory meals and the knowledge to integrate these practices into your daily life for lasting health benefits.

I invite you to continue with an open mind and a commitment to learning. I hope you will embrace this opportunity to change your diet. It can truly transform your life and the lives of those you love. Your first steps can start now.

Chapter 1

Inflammation's Link with Food

In the heart of a busy kitchen, where the crackle of a sizzling pan fills the air, cooking becomes more than just meal preparation; it's a meaningful act of self-care. Here, the fight against inflammation unfolds, not through dramatic acts, but through everyday decisions about what we serve on our plates and put into our bodies.

Acute or short-lived inflammation is the body's response to infection or injury, acting as a natural defense mechanism to protect and heal. However, when inflammation becomes chronic or long-lasting, it can serve as a silent driver of many health problems, including diabetes, heart disease, autoimmune disorders, and digestive issues.

Our food is one of the most powerful and often overlooked contributors to chronic inflammation. Our dietary choices can either fuel inflammation or help reduce it, making the connection between what we eat and our overall health more critical than ever.

This chapter discusses the intricate relationship between inflammation and diet to better understand how certain foods can trigger or calm the body's inflammatory response. Understanding this link is the first step toward harnessing the power of nutrition to support a healthier, more balanced body.

Decoding Your Body's Signal for Help

Inflammation is the body's natural alarm system, signaling that something is wrong. It's the physiological equivalent of a smoke alarm—a protective measure designed to safeguard our well-being. When we experience a cut on our finger or catch a cold, inflammation rushes in as the first responder, mobilizing our immune system to heal and defend. This acute inflammation is visible, tangible, and, most importantly, temporary, retreating once healing occurs.

However, when inflammation lingers, it becomes a silent saboteur, undermining health from beneath the surface. Chronic inflammation is a persistent activation of the immune response, operating under the radar and contributing to various diseases, from arthritis to heart disease and diabetes. The distinction between acute and chronic inflammation is crucial—not just in duration but also in its impact on our health. Acute inflammation is a chapter that closes; chronic inflammation is a book that never ends, continuously writing its narrative of damage unless we intervene.

The signs of chronic inflammation are often understated, whispering rather than shouting for attention. They manifest as fatigue that clings despite rest, unexplained joint pain, or a digestive system that rebels without warning. These symptoms, easy to dismiss as the wear and tear of life, are the body's subtle pleas for help, signaling the need to calm inflammation.

Food's Role in Health

The link between diet and inflammation is profound and deeply rooted in modern life. Our dietary choices, sedentary lifestyles, and persistent stressors significantly contribute to our body's inflammatory response.

Environmental exposure to pollutants and toxins also increases our body's inflammatory burden. Uniquely, diet not only contributes to the problem but also holds powerful potential as a solution.

The old wisdom of "you are what you eat" finds renewed importance here. Understanding the foods that worsen and those that calm inflammation is crucial as we adopt this new way of eating. Foods that provoke inflammation often masquerade as comfort foods or quick solutions for hunger. Identifying and choosing foods that alleviate inflammation over those that fuel it is transformative, shifting our diet from convenience to healing, where each meal choice is an act against chronic inflammation.

Principles and Practices of the Anti-Inflammatory Diet

Understanding how food affects inflammation allows us to make choices that nurture rather than harm our bodies. Following an anti-inflammatory diet is not about rigid rules but rather about making thoughtful, mindful decisions. The core principles of this diet emphasize whole, nutrient-dense foods that naturally reduce inflammation. Key elements include a variety of fruits and vegetables, whole grains, plant-based proteins like legumes and nuts, and healthy fats, especially those rich in omega-3 fatty acids. These foods provide essential nutrients that fight inflammation and promote overall health.

Hydration is often overlooked but plays a crucial role in reducing inflammation. Drinking enough water helps flush toxins from the body and keeps cells functioning optimally. Herbal teas and broths can also offer anti-inflammatory benefits. Reducing sugary drinks and alcohol further supports the body's detoxification and hydration processes.

Balancing macronutrients is another key aspect of the anti-inflammatory diet. Prioritizing complex carbohydrates, plant-based proteins, and healthy fats ensures a steady energy supply and reduces the risk of inflammation-triggering spikes in blood sugar. Processed carbohydrates and unhealthy fats should be avoided, as they contribute to inflammation and disrupt the body's balance. Nutrient-dense foods like fruits, vegetables, and nuts offer vitamins, minerals, and antioxidants that support the body's natural anti-inflammatory processes.

Portion control and meal timing are also important. Overeating, even healthy foods, can stress the digestive system and lead to inflammation. On the other hand, undereating can deprive the body of the nutrients it needs to fight inflammation. Eating smaller, balanced meals throughout the day can help stabilize blood sugar levels and provide consistent energy. This approach can be tailored to individual needs based on factors like activity levels, stress, and sleep patterns.

For example, an active person may require more calories and protein to support muscle repair and energy, while someone dealing with stress may need to focus on magnesium-rich foods and omega-3s to counteract the impact of stress hormones. By paying attention to portion sizes, meal timing, and macronutrient balance, the anti-inflammatory diet can be personalized to fit different lifestyles and health goals.

The Science Behind the Anti-Inflammatory Diet

Food plays a dual role in our body's metabolic functions—it can be a source of healing or, unintentionally, a trigger for damage. The foods we eat directly impact inflammation, making it essential to understand which foods help reduce it and which may cause harm. Certain ingredients, like trans fats found in processed foods, can raise LDL cholesterol and promote inflammation in the cardiovascular system. High-sugar diets and refined carbohydrates can lead to insulin resistance, a significant factor in inflammation. On the other hand, foods rich in omega-3 fatty acids, antioxidants, and phytonutrients can block inflammatory enzymes, neutralize free radicals, and protect cells from damage.

Gut health plays a central role in managing inflammation. A diet rich in fiber from plant-based foods supports the gut microbiome, a diverse community of microorganisms that help regulate inflammation. When fiber is metabolized by gut bacteria, it produces short-chain fatty acids (SCFAs) that have potent anti-inflammatory effects. A diet low in fiber and high in processed foods disrupts this balance, leading to issues like leaky gut syndrome, which can trigger widespread inflammation throughout the body.

The influence of the gut microbiome extends beyond digestion, affecting immune function, mental health, and overall well-being. A healthy gut supports immune system regulation and plays a role in producing neurotransmitters, which is evidence that gut health is linked to mood and mental clarity. By consuming anti-inflammatory foods that promote a healthy microbiome, we reduce inflammation and support broader aspects of our health, including mental well-being.

Growing scientific evidence supports the role of bioactive compounds in anti-inflammatory foods. These compounds reduce the risk of chronic diseases like heart disease, diabetes, and certain cancers. Omega-3 fatty acids, for example, have been shown to reduce heart disease risk, while the antioxidant resveratrol, found in grapes and red wine, has demonstrated anti-inflammatory and cancer-preventive properties.

Our food choices can also influence inflammation markers like C-reactive protein (CRP) and cytokines, including tumor necrosis factor-alpha (TNF-α) and interleukin-6 (IL-6). These markers are indicators of the levels of inflammation in the body. Research shows that diets rich in whole foods and low in processed items and added sugars can significantly lower CRP levels, reducing systemic or widespread inflammation.

Overall, the relationship between diet, inflammation, and health is complex but clear: the foods we choose profoundly affect our inflammatory status and overall well-being. Incorporating anti-inflammatory foods—rich in essential fatty acids, antioxidants, and other beneficial compounds—into our daily diet can reduce the risk of chronic diseases and improve our quality of life.

Identifying and Avoiding Inflammatory Foods

Minimizing inflammation through diet requires a careful approach, especially when navigating the complexities of modern food. Identifying which foods trigger inflammation is a personal process and can take time. Individuals react differently to certain foods based on their health conditions, genetics, allergies, or sensitivities. For example, while gluten and dairy may cause inflammation for some, others may not be bothered by them but find that nightshade vegetables, like tomatoes, eggplant, or even certain nuts, lead to inflammatory symptoms.

Customizing your anti-inflammatory diet involves experimentation. Many start by eliminating common inflammatory foods and then slowly reintroducing them to observe how their bodies respond. This trial-and-error approach helps create a personalized diet that minimizes inflammation while meeting individual health needs. Using a food and symptom tracker, like the one offered at the beginning of this book, can be invaluable during this process. Tracking what you eat and any symptoms that arise allows you to better understand how certain foods affect your body.

Understanding food labels is another crucial skill. Processed foods often contain additives, preservatives, and hidden sugars that contribute to inflammation. Ingredients like high fructose corn syrup, dextrose, and trans fats are often disguised under different names. Learning to decode labels will help you avoid these hidden inflammatory agents and make healthier choices. Ultra-processed foods are particularly problematic due to their high levels of refined grains, sugars, and unhealthy fats, all of which contribute to chronic inflammation. Although convenient, the long-term health costs of these foods make finding healthier alternatives essential.

Food sensitivities, which can subtly increase inflammation without obvious allergic reactions, are also worth considering. Identifying these sensitivities may require following an elimination diet. You can discover which foods exacerbate inflammation by removing the most common offenders and then slowly reintroducing them, one at a time. Though this process can be tedious and time-consuming, the resulting improvements in health and reduced inflammation are worth the effort.

Making practical diet swaps is a simple yet effective way to reduce inflammation. Replace refined grains with whole grains, choose lean proteins over processed meats, and add anti-inflammatory foods like berries, leafy greens, and fatty fish to your meals. These swaps support your health and offer an opportunity to explore new, flavorful foods. This approach isn't about restriction but about enriching your diet with nourishing and satisfying foods.

Avoiding inflammatory foods will become easier over time. This approach shifts the focus from what you're eliminating from your diet to what you're gaining—better health, more energy, and a clearer sense of well-being. Simple choices, like opting for a piece of fruit over a sugary snack or herbal tea instead of soda, help reduce inflammation and improve your overall health. Ultimately, this approach transforms eating into a conscious act of self-care.

Transitioning to an Anti-Inflammatory Diet

Transitioning to an anti-inflammatory diet is a gradual process that requires patience and commitment. Instead of overhauling your diet overnight, start with small, manageable changes. Begin by adding one anti-inflammatory food to each meal while slowly cutting back on processed foods.

For instance, you could include berries at breakfast, a salad with leafy greens at lunch, and a serving of fatty fish at dinner. As you incorporate more anti-inflammatory ingredients, the balance in your diet will naturally shift toward healthier choices.

Focus on achievable milestones. This transition is about progress, not perfection. It's important to remember that change takes time. Stay patient and open to exploring new foods and recipes that support an anti-inflammatory lifestyle.

Overcoming Challenges

Like any dietary change, shifting to an anti-inflammatory diet comes with its own set of challenges. Time constraints and food preferences can all create obstacles. The key is to view setbacks as part of the learning process, not as failures. Each challenge provides insight into what works and what doesn't, allowing you to fine-tune your approach.

Meal planning is essential for those with busy schedules. Setting aside time on the weekend to prepare meals in advance can help reduce stress during the week and ensure you stick to your anti-inflammatory goals. Batch cooking and freezing meals can save time and make it easier to avoid reaching for less healthy, processed options.

Creativity and flexibility are essential in households with varying dietary preferences. One option is to modify familiar recipes by swapping out inflammatory ingredients for healthier alternatives. Getting the whole family involved in meal planning and cooking may also be helpful. This can turn the endeavor into a shared experience rather than a solo effort.

By approaching these challenges with flexibility and a problem-solving mindset, you'll be better equipped to stay on track. Transitioning to an anti-inflammatory diet is not a race, and with persistence and adaptability, it's possible to overcome these and other hurdles and enjoy the long-term health benefits.

Dining Out and Social Occasions

Dining out and socializing are integral parts of life; sticking to an anti-inflammatory diet doesn't mean you have to miss out. With a bit of preparation and assertiveness, you can maintain your healthy eating habits while enjoying meals with friends, family, or colleagues. Navigating restaurant menus and social gatherings may present challenges, but with the right strategies, you can make informed choices that align with your dietary goals.

When dining out, doing a bit of research in advance is helpful. Many restaurants post their menus online so you can review the options before you arrive. This allows you to identify dishes that naturally align with an anti-inflammatory diet, such as grilled fish, salads, or vegetable-based entrees. Call the restaurant ahead to ask if they can prepare certain dishes using olive oil instead of vegetable oils or if they can accommodate any other dietary requests.

At the table, simple strategies like requesting dressings and sauces on the side give you more control over ingredients that may contain hidden sugars or unhealthy fats. Being mindful of portion sizes and focusing on whole, minimally processed foods will also help you stay on track without feeling deprived.

Social occasions often bring another layer of complexity, as peer pressure or limited food options can make it difficult to stick to your plan. Communicating your dietary needs clearly and confidently can help deflect unwanted pressure to indulge in foods that don't align with your goals. If you're concerned about the menu, eating a small, nutrient-dense snack before you go out can help curb temptation and ensure you aren't overly hungry when faced with fewer healthy options.

Alcohol, which can contribute to inflammation, requires moderation. If you choose to drink, opt for red wine, which contains resveratrol, or clear spirits mixed with low-sugar beverages. Alternating between alcoholic drinks and water helps you stay hydrated and reduces overall alcohol consumption.

For larger social events or gatherings, bringing a dish that fits your dietary needs ensures you can enjoy at least one option. This can help you stick to your goals and introduce others to the delicious possibilities of anti-inflammatory eating. With some planning, social dining becomes less of a challenge and more of an opportunity to share your healthy lifestyle with those around you. Dining with friends and family then becomes a shared experience that supports your well-being and relationships, ensuring you can stay on track without feeling restricted or left out.

Setting Realistic Goals

Setting realistic and achievable goals is key to long-term success when transitioning to an anti-inflammatory diet. As discussed previously in this chapter, start with small, manageable steps. Small changes allow you to build a sustainable routine without feeling overwhelmed.

Tracking your progress is a great way to stay motivated. Whether you use a journal, a mobile app, or even a note on your fridge, documenting your goals and accomplishments helps keep you accountable. Celebrating each achievement, no matter how small, reinforces positive behavior and keeps you focused on your health goals. This steady, gradual progress is far more sustainable than aiming for perfection right away.

Patience and persistence are essential in this process. This way of eating is about exploring new flavors, recipes, and habits that align with an anti-inflammatory lifestyle. As you introduce new ingredients and meal ideas, you'll develop a diet that supports your long-term health.

Incorporating Mindful Eating

Mindful eating can be a powerful tool as you adopt an anti-inflammatory diet. This practice involves being fully present while eating, paying attention to your body's hunger and fullness cues, and savoring each bite. Tuning into your body's signals can help you better differentiate between true hunger and emotional or habitual eating.

Engaging in mindful eating often leads to a more measured approach to meals. When you slow down and focus on the experience of eating, you're more likely to consume anti-inflammatory foods in appropriate portions and less likely to overeat. Mindful eating also enhances your enjoyment of food, allowing you to appreciate the textures, flavors, and nutrients that support your health.

This practice fosters a deeper connection to your body, helping you recognize how your food impacts your well-being. As you become more aware of how nourishing foods make you feel, your motivation to continue making anti-inflammatory choices will grow stronger. Over time, mindful eating becomes second nature, reinforcing your commitment to a healthier, inflammation-free lifestyle.

A Rewarding Transition

The transition to an anti-inflammatory diet is not just about changing what you eat—it's a self-directed move toward better health. It's about developing an awareness of the role diet plays in your overall well-being and adopting and benefiting from a healthier lifestyle.

Gradual transformation will occur as you set realistic goals, practice mindful eating, and embrace new flavors and foods. Through this step-by-step approach, the transition becomes manageable and rewarding, allowing you to explore the profound connection between diet and wellness. Each new food, each mindful meal, brings you closer to a healthier, more balanced life.

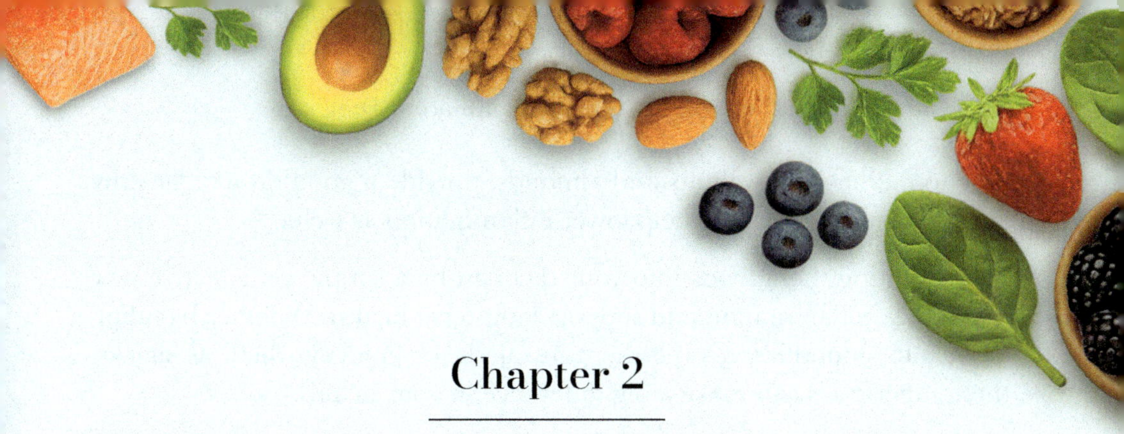

Chapter 2

Anti-Inflammatory Superfoods and Their Potent Powers

In the vibrant canvas of your kitchen, where colors burst from the chopping board and aromas swirl with promise, lies the key to unlocking the hidden power of nature's most potent ingredients: superfoods. These are the foods that nourish your body on a deeper level in the fight to calm inflammation.

The title of this chapter may conjure up visions of cape-wearing, crime-fighting fish, vegetables, and fruits. In reality, anti-inflammatory superfoods are a group of nutrient-rich foods known to reduce inflammation when eaten regularly. These foods are packed with healthy fats, antioxidants, vitamins, and minerals that work together to combat inflammation at the cellular level.

Common anti-inflammatory superfoods include fatty fish like salmon, which are rich in omega-3 fatty acids, known to lower inflammation markers in the body. Berries also make the list and are loaded with antioxidants like flavonoids, which help neutralize harmful free radicals. Other notable anti-inflammatory superfoods include leafy greens such as spinach and kale, high in vitamins A, C, and K. These vitamins are essential for reducing inflammation and supporting overall immune function. Nuts, like walnuts and almonds, provide a good dose of healthy fats and antioxidants that help lower inflammation as well.

Incorporating these foods into your diet can be a simple yet effective way to manage inflammation and support long-term health. Whether blending them into smoothies, tossing them in salads, or enjoying them as snacks, these superfoods can make a big difference in your health.

Omega-3 Fatty Acids from the Earth and Sea

Omega-3 fatty acids come from both seafood and plant sources. Fatty fish, like salmon, mackerel, and sardines, are some of the best options. If you're more into plant-based foods, flaxseeds, walnuts, and chia seeds are excellent sources, too.

Omega-3s are known for their anti-inflammatory properties. Specifically, EPA and DHA (from fish) and ALA (from plants) help reduce inflammation-related substances in the body, like eicosanoids and cytokines. These healthy fats can also improve heart health by lowering blood pressure, reducing triglycerides, and preventing arterial plaque. On top of that, omega-3s support brain health, potentially reducing the risk of depression and cognitive decline.

If you don't eat much fatty fish, you can still get your omega-3s through supplements. Fish oil supplements are rich in EPA and DHA, while algae-based supplements offer a plant-based alternative. When choosing a supplement, be sure to look for one tested for purity and potency.

Getting more omega-3s in your meals doesn't have to be complicated. Add a spoonful of flaxseed oil to your morning smoothie, or sprinkle chia seeds on your salad at lunch. Walnuts make a great snack alone, or you can add them to a homemade trail mix. Grilling a piece of salmon for dinner is a tasty way to boost your omega-3 intake. Simple additions like these help fight inflammation and keep your meals interesting and nutritious.

A Rainbow of Colorful Vegetables

Colorful vegetables are key players in fighting inflammation, and their vibrant colors actually indicate the presence of powerful anti-inflammatory compounds. Each color represents different antioxidants and phytonutrients that help your body reduce inflammation. For example, the reds and purples of vegetables like eggplants and bell peppers are rich in anthocyanins, which support heart health and help manage inflammation. Green vegetables contain lutein, which protects your eyes, while orange vegetables like carrots are high in beta-carotene, which supports your immune system and skin health.

Including 5-7 servings of colorful vegetables in your daily diet might sound like a lot, but it's easier than you think. It's not about completely changing what you eat. It's about adding more color and nutrition to your meals. A serving could be as simple as a half-cup of cooked vegetables or a cup of raw leafy greens added to your plate. The goal is to have a variety of colors in each meal, ensuring you're getting a wide range of nutrients that help calm inflammation and improve overall health.

How you cook your vegetables matters, too. While heat can make some nutrients more available, overcooking can lead to nutrient loss. Steaming is a gentle cooking method that preserves both nutrients and color, while sautéing with a bit of healthy oil can enhance the absorption of fat-soluble vitamins. Eating some vegetables raw, like bell peppers and carrots, can maximize their antioxidant content. Mixing up your cooking methods can keep things interesting in the kitchen and help you explore new flavors and textures.

Expanding your choices doesn't have to be intimidating. If you're used to sticking with just a few types of vegetables, you can start by swapping in more nutrient-dense options like spinach or kale in place of lettuce. Add a handful of spinach to a smoothie or some diced bell peppers to an omelet. For those feeling adventurous, ethnic markets offer a variety of less common vegetables, such as bitter melon or daikon radish, that can add new flavors and nutrients to your diet.

Getting kids or picky eaters to enjoy vegetables can be a challenge. Still, with a bit of creativity, it can be fun. Try a "rainbow challenge" where the goal is to eat a vegetable of every color throughout the week. You can also make eating vegetables more appealing by arranging them in fun shapes or blending them into smoothies where sweeter fruits mask the taste.

By incorporating a range of colorful vegetables into your meals, you're not just adding variety, but also boosting your body's ability to fight inflammation. Through thoughtful choices and preparation, these vegetables can become a vital part of your anti-inflammatory diet, helping you maintain better health from the inside out.

Nature's Pharmacy of Spices and Herbs

Spices and herbs aren't just for flavor—they're powerful tools for supporting your health, especially when fighting inflammation. This section dives into some of the most effective anti-inflammatory spices and herbs, like turmeric, ginger, and garlic, which have been valued for their healing properties for centuries.

Turmeric, known as 'Olena in Hawaiian, was among the "canoe crops" brought to the Hawaiian Islands by ancient Polynesian voyagers. These crops, essential for nutrition, medicine, and cultural practices, were carefully selected for their versatility and benefits.

Turmeric is especially valued for its bright yellow color and the compound curcumin, which is known to help reduce inflammation in the body. Curcumin has been shown to ease joint pain and swelling, making it particularly effective for managing conditions like arthritis. Today, turmeric continues to be celebrated for its healing properties. It is widely used to support joint health and overall well-being.

Ginger, another strong anti-inflammatory spice, contains gingerol, which helps reduce muscle pain and has antioxidant benefits. Garlic, famous for its bold taste and aroma, releases allicin when chopped or crushed—a compound that fights inflammation and boosts the immune system.

Knowing how to use and store spices and herbs is important. Examples include: combining turmeric with black pepper to enhance curcumin's absorption in the body, making it more effective; adding fresh herbs towards the end of cooking helps to preserve their flavor and benefits; and storing spices in airtight containers away from sunlight helps keep their potency for a longer period of time.

Healthy spices and herbs can be easily incorporated into your meals. Turmeric is excellent in curries, soups, and even in drinks like turmeric lattes. Ginger can be added to stir-fries, teas, or dressings, offering both flavor and health benefits. Garlic is incredibly versatile, adding depth to marinades, sauces, and sautés.

However, it is important to know how these powerful ingredients interact with certain medications. For instance, turmeric and ginger can act as blood thinners, so those on blood-thinning medications should use them cautiously. Garlic can also affect blood pressure and should be consumed in moderation if you're on medication for hypertension.

Incorporating these spices and herbs into your diet will enhance flavor and calm your inflammation. They help connect our food to our health, blending traditional wisdom with modern understanding. By adding them to your daily routine, you're making a simple yet powerful choice for your health.

The Powerful Benefits of Berries

Berries are more than just tasty snacks—they're potent allies in the fight against inflammation. These small, colorful fruits are packed with antioxidants like anthocyanins, quercetin, and vitamin C, which help protect your body from oxidative stress, a major contributor to inflammation and chronic diseases. Despite their small size, berries are nutritional powerhouses that offer a wide range of health benefits.

Different types of berries bring their own unique mix of vitamins, minerals, and phytochemicals to the table. Blueberries, for example, are rich in anthocyanins, giving them their deep blue color and providing strong anti-inflammatory and neuroprotective effects. Strawberries are high in manganese and vitamin C, which support heart health and reduce inflammation. Raspberries are loaded with dietary fiber, promoting gut health while also helping to fight inflammation. Blackberries are packed with vitamins C and K, fiber, and ellagic acid, making them excellent for combating oxidative stress.

When it comes to choosing between fresh and frozen berries, it's a common misconception that fresh is always better. In reality, frozen berries can be just as nutritious, if not more so, because they are often frozen at peak ripeness, preserving their antioxidants. Fresh berries can lose some of their nutrients during transportation and storage. In contrast, frozen berries retain most of their nutritional value. So frozen berries can offer a convenient and healthy option year-round. You can mix fresh and frozen berries into your diet for variety—fresh berries are great in cereals or salads, while frozen berries are perfect for smoothies or as a topping for yogurt.

Incorporating berries into your daily meals is easy and delicious. A morning smoothie made with mixed berries, spinach, and almond milk is a great way to start your day with an anti-inflammatory boost. A homemade trail mix with dried berries, nuts, and seeds makes a healthy mid-day snack. Berries can elevate any meal. A simple berry compote simmered with a touch of honey is perfect for topping whole-grain pancakes or oatmeal. Fresh berries can elevate a salad, adding a sweet contrast to the greens.

Berries may be small, but they can significantly impact your health. Adding them to your daily routine means you're not just enjoying their delicious flavor—you're making a conscious choice to support your health and well-being. Whether it's breakfast, a snack, or dessert, incorporating berries into your meals is an easy and enjoyable way to harness their anti-inflammatory power.

Nuts and Seeds as Your Crunchy Allies

Nuts and seeds seem like simple snacks, but they're actually powerful tools for managing inflammation. Packed with healthy fats, protein, and fiber, they're not just tasty but essential components of an anti-inflammatory diet. Despite their small size, nuts and seeds offer a wide range of benefits that can help keep inflammation in check and support overall health.

Each type of nut and seed has its own unique nutritional benefits. Almonds are rich in Vitamin E, an antioxidant that helps protect your cells from damage. Walnuts are high in omega-3 fatty acids, particularly alpha-linolenic acid (ALA), which is great for reducing inflammation. Chia seeds and flaxseeds are also excellent sources of ALA and fiber, making them great choices for boosting your intake of anti-inflammatory nutrients. Choosing a variety of nuts and seeds is a smart way to get a broad spectrum of health benefits.

However, it's important to be mindful of portion sizes when it comes to nuts and seeds because they are calorie-dense. A small handful, about an ounce, can easily contain around 160 calories, depending on the type. While they're incredibly nutritious, it's easy to overdo it. The key is moderation—enjoying nuts and seeds in a way that adds to your diet without overwhelming it.

Nuts and seeds are also incredibly versatile in the kitchen, making it easy to incorporate them into your meals throughout the day. They're great for adding crunch and flavor to salads or for sprinkling over breakfast bowls and baked goods. You can even use them in dressings and sauces, where almonds or cashews can add a creamy texture without the need for dairy. Their adaptability means you can enjoy the nutritional benefits of nuts and seeds in a variety of delicious ways.

The rich nutritional profiles of nuts and seeds offer significant benefits when consumed in moderation, and their versatility makes them easy to enjoy in many different dishes. Whether snacking on them or using them as a key ingredient in your meals, nuts and seeds are valuable allies in maintaining an anti-inflammatory lifestyle.

The Role of Probiotics and Prebiotics

The health of our gut microbiome plays a critical role in managing inflammation and overall well-being. This community of beneficial bacteria in our digestive system influences many aspects of our health, including how our body responds to inflammation. A balanced and thriving gut microbiome is essential for keeping inflammation in check and maintaining harmony within our bodies.

Probiotics, which are the beneficial bacteria found in foods like yogurt, kefir, sauerkraut, and kimchi, are key players in supporting gut health. By regularly consuming these foods, we help strengthen our gut's defenses, making it harder for harmful substances to trigger inflammation. Each serving of probiotic-rich food contributes to building a strong microbiome that can effectively manage inflammatory responses.

But probiotics alone aren't enough—they need nourishment to thrive, and that's where prebiotics come in. Prebiotics are non-digestible fibers found in foods like onions, garlic, bananas, asparagus, and whole grains. These fibers ferment in the gut, providing the fuel that probiotics need to grow and flourish. Together, probiotics and prebiotics work in harmony to create a healthy gut environment that supports overall health and reduces inflammation.

Supporting gut health requires more than just adding a few specific foods to your diet; it's about embracing a diverse and balanced approach to eating. Regularly incorporating various probiotic and prebiotic foods into your meals can help ensure that your gut microbiome remains robust and resilient. For example, starting your day with a breakfast that includes whole-grain cereal, bananas, and yogurt is an easy way to include both prebiotics and probiotics. Adding fermented vegetables as a side dish to meals or enjoying a kefir smoothie as a snack are other simple yet effective ways to support your gut.

Variety is key to maintaining a healthy gut microbiome. Experimenting with different probiotic and prebiotic foods keeps your meals exciting and ensures that your gut receives the broad spectrum of nutrients it needs to stay healthy.

Focusing on gut health through the strategic use of probiotics and prebiotics can directly influence our body's inflammatory responses. This approach highlights the deep connection between what we eat and how our bodies function. Nurturing our gut microbiome is more than just supporting digestion; it's crucial to defending against inflammation and maintaining overall health. This dietary strategy reinforces the idea that the food we eat has the power to heal, making gut health a fundamental aspect of any anti-inflammatory journey.

Keeping Inflammation Under Control

As we continue to explore the impact of diet on inflammation, the importance of anti-inflammatory superfoods becomes clear. These amazing powerhouses, incorporated into a thoughtful diet, can significantly enhance our well-being by helping keep inflammation under control. Prioritizing gut health is a simple yet powerful way to take care of our bodies, demonstrating the profound influence that our food choices have on our health. By making mindful decisions about what we eat, we can support our gut, reduce inflammation, and ultimately improve our quality of life.

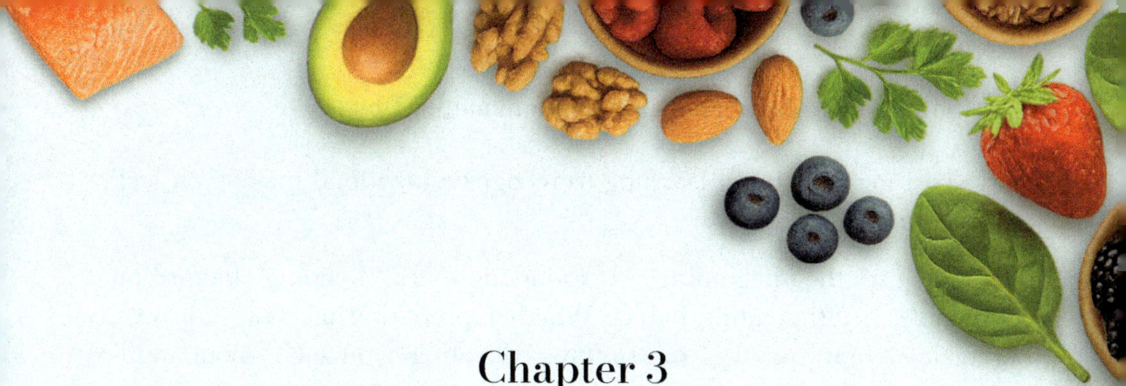

Chapter 3

Starting Your Anti-Inflammatory Diet

At the break of dawn, when the world is a quiet murmur and the day stretches ahead untouched, the decisions we make can set the tone for the hours to come. In these early moments, the choice of what to fuel our bodies with becomes not just a matter of routine but a declaration of how we wish to live.

Preparation is an essential aspect of transitioning to an anti-inflammatory way of eating. Before you dive in, taking time to plan and organize can make the process smoother and more sustainable. Once you've familiarized yourself with the diet's core principles, stocking your kitchen with the right tools and ingredients is the next step.

Creating detailed meal plans and shopping lists ensures you have everything you need to get started, reducing the temptation to fall back on unhealthy choices. Clearing out processed, inflammatory foods and replacing them with nutrient-dense, whole foods sets the stage for success.

Each meal and ingredient plays a part in the early stages of adopting the anti-inflammatory way of eating. This time is about discovering what works best for your body, learning to recognize how food makes you feel, and adjusting accordingly.

This is just the beginning—a foundation for building long-term, sustainable, healthy eating habits. Whether preparing meals in advance, organizing your pantry, or simply educating yourself about anti-inflammatory foods, the more groundwork you lay before you begin, the more confident and empowered you'll feel as you embrace this new way of eating.

Early Days of Your New Lifestyle

Planning a week of meals that support an anti-inflammatory lifestyle requires some thought. Still, it doesn't have to be complicated. The goal is to prepare breakfasts that are easy to make, lunches that keep you going, dinners that are comforting, and snacks that won't derail your progress, all while fitting it into a busy schedule.

With your weekly meal plan in hand, a shopping list based on your food choices assures you have all the ingredients you need to prepare your healthy meals. Group your items on your shopping list by category—like produce, proteins, and grains—to make shopping quicker and easier. This list will help you stay focused, ensuring you don't miss anything essential while avoiding unnecessary or unhealthy purchases.

Batch cooking is another great strategy for staying on track during the week. Dedicate a couple of hours over the weekend to cook essential ingredients like grains, proteins, and vegetables. These staples can then be mixed and matched into different meals. For example, you can use cooked quinoa in breakfast bowls, salads, or as a side dish. Roasted vegetables can be added to pastas or served with grilled proteins. This advanced preparation saves time during the week and makes healthy eating more accessible.

Freezing meals is also a helpful way to ensure you always have nutritious options ready to go. Soups, stews, and casseroles freeze well. A quick reheat of pre-prepared meals can be especially useful on busy days when you don't have time to cook and will help you avoid reaching for less healthy options.

Repurposing leftovers can also save time and effort. For example, you can turn last night's dinner into today's lunch with minimal effort—like using roasted chicken from dinner in a salad for lunch. This can reduce food waste while keeping your meals interesting and varied throughout the week.

With a bit of planning, meal prep, and creativity, following an anti-inflammatory diet can fit seamlessly into your life. Weekly planning, smart shopping, batch cooking, freezing meals, and using leftovers contribute to making healthy eating a sustainable habit.

Shopping Strategies and Budget-Friendly Tips for Whole Foods

Shopping for an anti-inflammatory diet requires a thoughtful approach, but it doesn't need to be expensive. You can nourish your body without breaking the bank by focusing on buying in bulk, using seasonal foods, and making smart choices about organic produce.

Bulk buying is another great way to save money, especially for pantry staples like grains, beans, nuts, and seeds. These ingredients are key components of an anti-inflammatory diet and can have long shelf lives. Just make sure to keep them in airtight containers to preserve freshness, and store items like nuts and seeds in the fridge or freezer to prevent spoilage.

Buying seasonal fruits and vegetables is one of the best ways to get fresh, nutritious food at an affordable price. Seasonal produce is often cheaper because it doesn't have to travel as far, and it's at its peak in terms of availability, flavor, and nutritional value. Eating seasonally also gives your diet variety throughout the year, whether it's berries in the summer, leafy greens in the winter, or root vegetables in the fall.

Because seasonal produce is only available for a limited time, preserving techniques like freezing, canning, and fermenting help us enjoy its benefits year-round. Freezing fruits and vegetables at their peak retains their nutrients, allowing us to enjoy the flavors of summer in winter. Canning transforms tomatoes, cucumbers, and berries into sauces, pickles, and jams, while fermentation creates probiotic-rich foods like sauerkraut and kimchi that support gut health. These methods capture the flavors and nutrients of each season, extending the bounty and offering variety even when fresh options are limited.

Shopping at farmers' markets or joining a Community Supported Agriculture (CSA) program are other ways to find fresh, local produce at a reasonable price. These options often give you access to a wider variety of seasonal fruits and vegetables than a regular grocery store, and you're supporting local farmers in the process. CSAs provide weekly shares of fresh produce throughout the growing season, encouraging you to cook with a variety of seasonal ingredients. You can find CSAs and local Farmer's Markets by accessing the free website: **LocalHarvest.org** and searching by zip code or city.

The choice to buy organic produce can result in higher grocery bills, but when is it necessary? That question can be answered by consulting the lists provided by the Environmental Working Group (EWG). These lists, known as the "Dirty Dozen" and the "Clean Fifteen," are updated annually. The "Dirty Dozen" lists fruits and vegetables with the highest pesticide levels. The "Clean Fifteen" features produce with the lowest levels of pesticides, so buying non-organic is usually fine.

These lists provide information that can help you decide when to spend the extra money and buy the organic options for specific fruits and vegetables, based on your preferences and budget. This approach can help you make healthier choices without overspending. Here are the latest lists from the EWG, based on their analysis of pesticide residue levels on fruits and vegetables, as of this writing.

Dirty Dozen (2024)

The **Dirty Dozen** includes fruits and vegetables that have been found to have the highest levels of pesticide residues. Whenever possible, buy organic options for these products.

Dirty Dozen 2024		
1. Strawberries	5. Peaches	9. Bell Peppers
2. Spinach	6. Pears	10. Cherries
3. Kale, Collard, & Mustard Greens	7. Nectarines	11. Blueberries
4. Grapes	8. Apples	12. Green Beans

Clean Fifteen (2024)

The **Clean Fifteen** includes produce that generally has the least pesticide residue, so saving your money and buying the non-organic option is usually fine.

Clean Fifteen 2024		
1. Carrots	6. Cabbage	11. Papaya
2. Sweet Potatoes	7. Kiwi	12. Onions
3. Mangoes	8. Honeydew Melon	13. Pineapple
4. Mushrooms	9. Asparagus	14. Sweet Corn
5. Watermelon	10. Sweet Peas (Frozen)	15. Avocados

Incorporating these shopping strategies—buying seasonal produce, purchasing in bulk, exploring farmers' markets, and using the EWG guides—helps you follow an anti-inflammatory diet in a way that's both affordable and sustainable. It also connects you more deeply to the food you eat, fostering healthier habits that support your well-being and the environment.

Review Labels for Hidden Inflammatory Ingredients

Shopping for groceries can be tricky, especially when navigating the abundance of packaged foods that often hide inflammatory ingredients behind vague or misleading labels. Even products marketed as healthy can contain ingredients that contribute to inflammation. The key is learning to read labels carefully and recognize the ingredients that are not as healthy as they seem.

Added sugar is a common hidden culprit that can appear under many different names. Besides the usual "sugar," you might see ingredients like high fructose corn syrup, dextrose, sucrose, agave nectar, and maltose. When consumed in excess, these sweeteners can contribute to inflammation. Be mindful of ingredient lists to make sure these sugars aren't sneaking into foods that seem otherwise healthy, like granola bars, yogurt, or sauces.

Unhealthy fats, especially trans fats, are another group to watch for. These are often found in foods like baked goods, margarine, and processed snacks. Trans fats may appear on labels as "partially hydrogenated oils." Even if a product claims to have "0 grams of trans fat," it may still contain small amounts if each serving has less than 0.5 grams. That means you could unknowingly consume trans fats if you're not checking the ingredient list carefully.

Artificial additives like preservatives, colorings, and flavor enhancers also lurk in processed foods. Ingredients like sodium nitrite (used in processed meats), artificial colors (such as Red 40 and Yellow 5), and flavor enhancers like monosodium glutamate (MSG) can trigger inflammation in some people. These additives are commonly found in foods like snack chips, deli meats, and frozen meals. Opt for whole, minimally processed foods with simple ingredient lists you can easily understand whenever possible.

The goal is to eat clean, which means choosing foods with ingredients that are as close to their natural state as possible. Focus on foods like whole grains, fresh vegetables, lean proteins, and healthy fats. Shop the outer aisles of the grocery store, where fresh produce, grains, and refrigerated goods are typically found, and avoid the highly processed options in the center aisles.

Switching to a diet rich in whole foods doesn't mean giving up flavor or convenience. There are plenty of healthier versions of familiar foods. For example, whole-grain bread and pasta offer more nutrients and fiber than refined versions. Snacks like air-popped popcorn or raw nuts provide a satisfying crunch without unhealthy fats or artificial additives. Sweet treats can be healthier when made with natural sweeteners like honey, dates, or maple syrup rather than processed sugars.

Reading labels isn't just about avoiding hidden ingredients—it's about making empowered choices for your health. Once you learn how to spot these inflammatory agents, you can shop with confidence, avoiding foods that inflame and choosing foods that calm inflammation.

The Essential Anti-Inflammatory Kitchen Toolkit

Creating an anti-inflammatory kitchen starts with having the right tools and ingredients on hand to make preparing healthy meals easier and more enjoyable. A well-stocked kitchen can help you consistently cook meals that support your health without feeling overwhelmed.

Key tools for an anti-inflammatory kitchen include:

- **High-powered blender**: Great for smoothies, soups, and sauces, a blender makes it easy to add nutrient-dense foods like leafy greens, fruits, and seeds to your diet.
- **Food Processor:** This handy tool can make chopping and preparing vegetables a breeze, freeing up precious time for other things.
- **Slow cooker or pressure cooker**: These tools are perfect for making soups, stews, and other meals that require little hands-on time. You can prepare meals in bulk to freeze or prep for the week, and they'll be ready when you need them.
- **Quality knives and cutting boards**: Good knives make chopping fruits and vegetables quicker and more efficient, and a

sturdy cutting board gives you the surface you need for meal prep.

- **Non-stick or stainless-steel pans**: These pans allow you to cook with less oil while still delivering delicious results. They're ideal for sautéing vegetables or cooking lean proteins.
- **Glass storage containers**: These are useful for storing prepped ingredients or leftovers, keeping food fresh and reducing waste.

With the right kitchen tools, you can set yourself up for success when it comes to following an anti-inflammatory diet. It becomes easier to cook meals at home, control ingredients, and avoid the hidden inflammatory ingredients found in processed foods.

Pantry Staples

Having a well-stocked pantry is key to sticking with an anti-inflammatory diet. Whole grains like quinoa and brown rice provide a hearty base for meals, rich in fiber and essential nutrients that support gut health and reduce inflammation. Keep a variety of legumes, such as lentils, chickpeas, and black beans, on hand for plant-based protein options that are versatile enough to use in soups, salads, and side dishes. Extra virgin olive oil, known for its heart-healthy fats and anti-inflammatory properties, should always be within reach for cooking and dressing salads. Coconut milk is another staple, perfect for adding creaminess to curries, soups, and smoothies.

Nuts and seeds are also important pantry staples—almonds, walnuts, chia seeds, and flaxseeds are rich in omega-3 fatty acids and fiber. Stock up on natural almond and peanut butter, as well as tahini, for easy snacks and homemade sauces or dressings. These ingredients serve as the foundation for a variety of healthy meals. With the proper pantry setup, you'll always be ready to whip up an anti-inflammatory dish with minimal effort.

Spices and Herbs

Spices and herbs enhance the flavor of your meals and offer numerous health benefits, including anti-inflammatory properties. With its active ingredient, curcumin, turmeric is one of the most powerful anti-inflammatory spices. It can be added to soups, stews, and teas. Ginger is another go-to for reducing inflammation, and its zesty flavor works well in stir-fries, smoothies, and herbal teas. Cinnamon is great for adding sweetness to dishes while helping to regulate blood sugar levels, which can influence inflammation.

Fresh herbs like basil, cilantro, and parsley bring bright flavors and a boost of antioxidants to salads, sauces, and garnishes. Dried herbs such as oregano and thyme are excellent for seasoning meats and vegetables, and they're loaded with compounds that reduce oxidative stress. Having a variety of spices and herbs on hand allows you to experiment with flavors while also supporting your health.

Storage and Organization

Keeping your kitchen organized is essential for easy meal prep and making the most of your anti-inflammatory ingredients. Store grains, nuts, seeds, and legumes in glass jars with clear labels so you can quickly see what you have and what needs restocking. Organize your spices in racks with labels facing outward for easy access so you can find what you need without rummaging through cabinets.

In the fridge, use bins or containers to organize fresh produce, ensuring vegetables and fruits are easy to grab and use in your daily meals. This type of organization makes cooking more enjoyable and reduces stress, as everything you need is at your fingertips. A well-organized kitchen encourages creativity and makes sticking to your healthy eating plan easier.

Understanding Food Intolerances and Allergies

Dealing with food intolerances and allergies requires a combination of self-awareness and knowledge. Understanding how your body reacts to certain foods is essential for anyone adopting an anti-inflammatory diet. This process can be challenging, but it's a crucial step toward finding the right foods that nourish your body without causing harm. By learning to recognize how your body responds to different foods, you can develop a diet that supports your health and reduces inflammation.

Food intolerances, which are less severe than allergies but still impactful, can manifest in various ways, such as digestive issues, skin problems, fatigue, or headaches. Common triggers include dairy, gluten, soy, and certain nuts. It's important to pay attention to how you feel after eating specific foods. By connecting your symptoms to what you've eaten, you can begin to identify patterns that point to potential intolerances.

As previously discussed, an elimination diet is a helpful tool in this process. This method involves removing suspected trigger foods from your diet for a period of time and then reintroducing them one at a time to observe any reactions. Although this approach takes patience, it provides valuable insights into which foods may be contributing to inflammation and discomfort. By systematically eliminating and reintroducing foods, you can create a diet that better aligns with your body's needs, reducing symptoms and improving overall well-being.

Food allergies, on the other hand, often cause more immediate and severe reactions. When your body reacts to an allergen, it can trigger symptoms ranging from mild discomfort to life-threatening anaphylaxis. For those with specific food allergies, avoiding these foods entirely is crucial. That means diligently reading food labels to avoid hidden allergens and being cautious when eating out. Fortunately, many alternative ingredients are available, allowing you to enjoy a wide variety of foods without risking an allergic reaction.

Working with healthcare professionals like dietitians or allergists can benefit those with food intolerances and allergies. These healthcare professionals can help you identify specific triggers, provide guidance on managing your diet, and ensure you're meeting your nutritional needs. With their support, you can confidently manage food sensitivities and allergies while following an anti-inflammatory eating plan.

Crafting Your Anti-Inflammatory Way of Eating

Understanding your body's unique relationship with food allows you to make informed choices that promote health and reduce inflammation. This personalized approach is empowering and essential to crafting a way of eating that works for you. By listening to your body and seeking expert guidance when needed, you can move forward with a clearer understanding of what foods serve you best.

With this knowledge, you're ready to fully embrace the transformative potential of anti-inflammatory foods and learn how to seamlessly integrate them into your everyday meals.

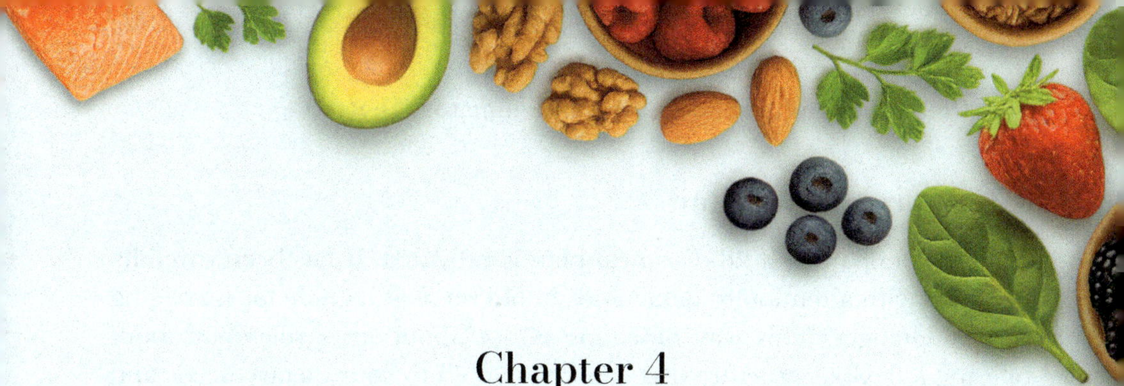

Chapter 4

Meal Planning for a Successful Transition

In the quiet moments before a meal, when the day's demands are set aside, the art of creating a meal unfolds without hurry or stress. Here, stress-free meal plans take shape—designed not just to nourish but to simplify, to offer a sense of ease amidst the chaos of the day.

When it comes to meal planning, preparation is critical to success. You may have heard the famous quote by Benjamin Franklin, "If you fail to plan, you are planning to fail." This is especially true when transitioning to a new way of eating, such as an anti-inflammatory diet. A well-thought-out meal plan provides a clear guide for the week ahead, helping you stay organized and motivated as you adjust to your new food choices. Outlining meals, snacks, and hydration goals gives you structure while keeping you on track toward your health goals.

A Comprehensive Plan

In the next chapter, a 28-day meal plan is provided. It has been carefully designed with attention to detail and should serve as a guide for managing dietary changes. This way of eating is not about strict rules but about offering a flexible structure that can be adapted to your dietary needs and your daily routine. Feel free to make any necessary changes in accordance with your preferences and your sensitivities, if known.

For breakfast, you might choose a simple option like avocado toast, packed with healthy fats and fiber, or go for something more substantial like a spinach and mushroom omelet, filled with protein and essential nutrients. Lunches could vary from a light quinoa and chickpea salad with lemon-tahini dressing to a filling vegetable soup with a side of whole-grain bread. Dinners give you a chance to relax and enjoy flavorful dishes like grilled salmon with roasted Brussels sprouts and sweet potatoes or a hearty lentil stew simmered with turmeric, carrots, and kale. Snacks are also on the menu to keep your energy steady, with options like apple slices with almond butter or fresh veggies with hummus.

Weekly Shopping Lists

To simplify your grocery shopping, detailed weekly shopping lists have been included. These lists are organized by category, such as produce, proteins, and pantry staples, to make your shopping efficient and stress-free.

With everything laid out, you'll avoid unnecessary purchases and ensure you have all the ingredients needed for the week. This approach saves time and encourages mindful food choices, helping you feel more connected to the meals you're preparing and the ingredients you're using. Just remember to adjust your shopping lists if you choose to make any changes or substitutions in your meal plan.

Adapting Recipes for Dietary Restrictions

When following an anti-inflammatory diet, adapting recipes to fit individual dietary restrictions becomes an opportunity to get creative and personalize meals. Instead of viewing food sensitivities as obstacles, they provide a chance to explore new ingredients and techniques that make eating enjoyable.

You can still have delicious meals that help reduce inflammation by making adjustments to ingredients. For instance, if a recipe calls for nuts but a person who will be eating the meal has an allergy, seeds can easily be swapped in, or the ingredient can be eliminated.

For those watching their carb intake, high-carb dishes can be balanced with low-carb alternatives. This flexibility makes the meal plan a valuable tool for a wide range of individuals, ensuring that it can be tailored to fit personal needs while supporting healthy eating.

Cultural Variations

Understanding that food preferences are shaped by culture, the meal plan includes adaptations that honor diverse culinary traditions. A classic Western breakfast of eggs and toast can be transformed with a Mexican twist by adding black beans, avocado, and salsa. A simple salad can be enhanced with Mediterranean flavors like olives, feta, and za'atar. These cultural variations add variety to the meal plan and celebrate the global influences that make our meals more exciting and enjoyable.

Gluten-Free and Dairy-Free Alternatives

For those with gluten or dairy sensitivities, adapting recipes means finding alternative ingredients that maintain the flavor and texture of the original dish. Gluten-free options like almond flour, buckwheat flour, or gluten-free oat flour can replace wheat flour, offering a solution and introducing richer, more complex flavors to your meals. Whether in baked goods or sauces, these substitutes add nutrition and variety to your diet.

Dairy-free alternatives are equally versatile. Coconut milk or almond milk can replace cream, while cashew cheese or nutritional yeast can substitute for traditional cheese in many dishes. These swaps provide creamy textures and full-bodied flavors without the inflammatory effects that some people experience with dairy. By using these ingredients, you can enjoy your favorite dishes while supporting your health.

Vegetarian and Vegan Adaptations

Options for adapting recipes for those following vegetarian and vegan diets involve using plant-based protein sources. Legumes, tofu, tempeh, and lentils are excellent protein alternatives to meat. They can be incorporated into stir-fries, salads, or stews. These options are nutrient-dense and provide a satisfying base for many meals.

Nutritional yeast, a popular ingredient in vegan cooking, offers a savory, cheesy flavor and is rich in B vitamins. Combined with other umami-rich ingredients like mushrooms or tomatoes, it can help build deep, satisfying flavors in plant-based dishes. The key to creating fulfilling vegetarian or vegan meals is layering flavors with herbs, spices, and healthy fats to make each dish both delicious and nourishing.

The Low-FODMAP Diet

The acronym **FODMAP** stands for **Fermentable Oligosaccharides, Disaccharides, Monosaccharides, and Polyols**. These short-chain carbohydrates can be poorly absorbed in the small intestine, leading to fermentation by gut bacteria. For some people, especially those with irritable bowel syndrome (IBS) or other digestive disorders, this fermentation can cause symptoms like bloating, gas, abdominal pain, and diarrhea.

Here's a breakdown of what each part of the acronym means:

- **Fermentable**: Refers to the process where gut bacteria ferment these carbohydrates, producing gas and bloating.
- **Oligosaccharides**: Found in foods like wheat, rye, onions, and garlic. They include fructans and galacto-oligosaccharides.
- **Disaccharides**: The main disaccharide in the FODMAP group is lactose, found in dairy products like milk, soft cheeses, and yogurt.

- **Monosaccharides**: This primarily refers to fructose, found in foods like honey, apples, and high-fructose corn syrup.
- **Polyols**: Sugar alcohols such as sorbitol and mannitol, found in some fruits (like stone fruits) and artificial sweeteners.

The low-FODMAP diet focuses on reducing or eliminating foods high in these specific carbohydrates to alleviate digestive symptoms. It is often recommended for individuals with IBS or gut sensitivities to follow a low-FODMAP diet. Adapting recipes for this diet involves replacing high-FODMAP foods with alternatives that are easier on the digestive system. For example, using the green parts of spring onions instead of regular onions or incorporating garlic-infused olive oil can maintain flavor without triggering discomfort.

These small but thoughtful adjustments allow those following a low-FODMAP diet to enjoy a wide variety of dishes. By focusing on ingredients that soothe rather than aggravate the gut, meals can still be flavorful and satisfying while promoting better digestive health.

Customization Tips

Customizing recipes to fit your dietary needs empowers you to take control of your health. Understanding how ingredients work in a recipe allows you to make substitutions without losing the essence of the dish. For example, replacing eggs in baking with a flaxseed or chia seed mixture can work for those with egg allergies or on a vegan diet. Similarly, using blended cashews or cauliflower in soups can replicate the creaminess of dairy-based versions.

Customization encourages experimentation. Sometimes, a substitution slightly alters the dish, but this can lead to delightful new flavors and textures. This flexibility invites you to move beyond strict recipes and trust your instincts in the kitchen, creating a deeper connection with the food you prepare. By being open to adjustments, you turn cooking into a mindful, creative experience that supports your health goals and personal preferences.

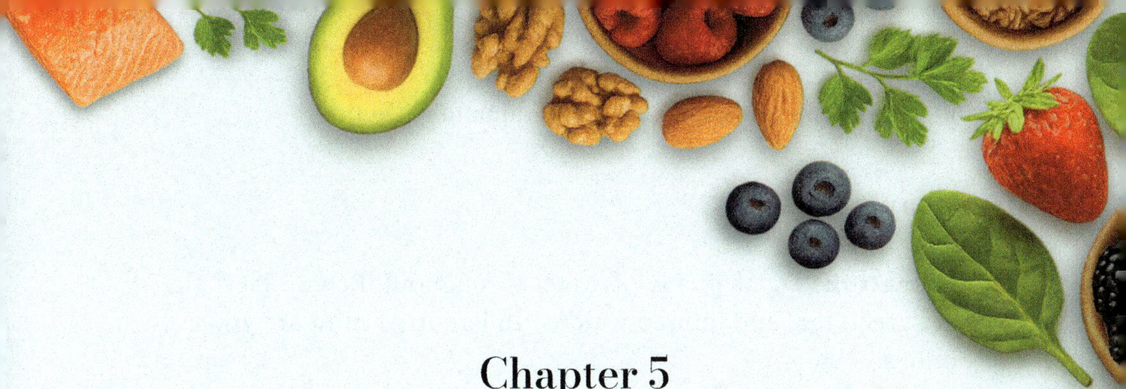

Chapter 5

28-Day Stress-Free Meal Plan

A thoughtfully crafted meal plan marks the beginning of a quiet transformation—not in sweeping changes, but in the deliberate choices made one ingredient, one meal at a time. It gently guides with clear, practical steps, mindful of the busy rhythms of everyday life.

This 4-week meal plan is designed to provide ease and variety while emphasizing whole, anti-inflammatory ingredients to support your health and well-being. It offers flexibility, allowing you to swap in seasonal vegetables and your preferred proteins to suit your taste and dietary needs.

Daily snacks can also be customized with a range of fruit and vegetable options, making the plan adaptable and enjoyable. Visiting local Farmer's Markets is encouraged to incorporate fresh, seasonal produce into your meals and snacks, adding both flavor and nutritional value. Remember to adjust your shopping list accordingly to reflect any changes you make, ensuring your kitchen is always stocked with the essentials needed for success.

Meal Plan Tips:

- **Hydration:** Drink plenty of water throughout the day. Herbal teas, green tea, and infused water with lemon or mint are great options.
- **Meal Prep:** Preparing meals or ingredients (like overnight oats, chopped veggies, and pre-cooked grains like quinoa and brown rice) can save time during the week.
- **Spices:** Incorporate anti-inflammatory spices like turmeric, ginger, and garlic, or the anti-inflammatory spice blend, into your meals to boost flavor and health benefits.
- **Portion Control:** Adjust portion sizes based on your hunger and nutritional needs.
- **Substitutions:** As discussed, you can substitute fruits, vegetables, proteins (e.g., chicken with tofu, or vice versa), or grains (e.g., quinoa with brown rice) to suit your preferences and food tolerances.

28-Day Meal Plan

This comprehensive anti-inflammatory meal plan is flexible and easy to follow, designed to guide you through a month of balanced and nourishing meals. With breakfast, lunch, dinner, and two snacks provided daily, it helps you maintain steady energy levels, reduce inflammation, and curb unhealthy cravings. The focus is on whole, nutrient-rich ingredients, including colorful vegetables, lean proteins, healthy fats, and antioxidant-packed fruits. Each meal is crafted to be as simple to prepare as it is flavorful, making it easy to stay consistent. Recipes for each meal and snack are included in the chapters that follow, offering variety while helping you develop lasting, healthy habits.

Coordinated Shopping Lists

To make meal preparation easier, this plan includes weekly shopping lists that align with the recipes for each week. These lists are carefully organized to reduce stress and streamline your trips to the grocery store.

By having all ingredients planned in advance, you can focus on enjoying the cooking process and nourishing your body without worrying about missing essentials. The lists are adaptable, so if you decide to substitute or adjust recipes to suit your preferences or seasonal availability, you can update your shopping list accordingly.

Each list is built around whole, fresh ingredients and pantry staples to support anti-inflammatory eating. By sticking to the lists, you'll ensure you have all the tools needed to prepare meals that are not only nutritious but also full of flavor. These shopping lists encourage you to explore local markets for fresh, seasonal produce and to keep your pantry stocked with versatile essentials like olive oil, herbs, and spices. This thoughtful approach to grocery shopping helps set you up for success, making it easier to embrace this 28-day plan and integrate its principles into your everyday routine.

Meal Plan - Week 1: Off to a Great Start

Day	Meal	Recipe Name
Day 1	**Breakfast**	Smoothie with Spinach, Pineapple, Ginger, and Flaxseed
	Snack 1	Sliced Apple with Almond Butter
	Lunch	Quinoa and Chickpea Salad with Lemon-Tahini Dressing
	Snack 2	Carrot and Celery Sticks with Hummus
	Dinner	Sheet-Pan Salmon with Veggies
Day 2	**Breakfast**	Chia Seed Pudding - Mango, Coconut Milk, Pistachios
	Snack 1	Mixed Nuts
	Lunch	Lentil and Vegetable Soup
	Snack 2	Cucumber Slices with Guacamole
	Dinner	Grilled Chicken with Sautéed Spinach and Brown Rice
Day 3	**Breakfast**	Smoked Salmon & Avocado Breakfast Bowl with Capers
	Snack 1	Bell Peppers with Tzatziki Dip
	Lunch	Sweet Potato and Black Bean Tacos
	Snack 2	Fresh Pineapple Chunks
	Dinner	Stir-Fried Tofu with Vegetables over Quinoa
Day 4	**Breakfast**	Quinoa Bowl with Coconut, Berries, and Almond Butter
	Snack 1	Sliced Pear with Walnuts
	Lunch	Tuna Salad with Olive Oil and Fresh Herbs
	Snack 2	Fresh Berrries
	Dinner	Turkey Chili
Day 5	**Breakfast**	Greek Yogurt Parfait (with Strawberries and Walnuts)
	Snack 1	Orange Slices and Almonds
	Lunch	Avocado and Hummus Veggie Wrap
	Snack 2	Sliced Radishes and Cucumbers with Hummus
	Dinner	Baked Cod with Roasted Brussels Sprouts and Quinoa
Day 6	**Breakfast**	Scrambled Eggs - Spinach, Tomatoes, & Avocado Toast
	Snack 1	Smoothie - Spinach, Mango, Pineapple, and Chia Seeds
	Lunch	Roasted Chickpea, Quinoa, and Veggie Bowl
	Snack 2	Sliced Bell Peppers and Cherry Tomatoes
	Dinner	Zucchini Noodles with Pesto and Cherry Tomatoes
Day 7	**Breakfast**	Chia Seed Pudding with Coconut Milk and Mango
	Snack 1	Watermelon Slices and Pumpkin Seeds
	Lunch	Chicken and Avocado Salad
	Snack 2	Dark Chocolate Square and Green Tea
	Dinner	Baked Chicken Breasts with Root Vegetables & Brown Rice

Shopping List - Week 1

Produce:	Proteins, Refrigerator, and Pantry:
Leafy Greens: 7 cups spinach 1 cup mixed greens **Vegetables:** 3 bell peppers 2 medium zucchinis 12 oz cherry tomatoes 2 medium sweet potatoes 8 oz Brussels sprouts 1 small onion (color of your choice) 1 small red onion 2 carrots 1 celery stalk 1 cucumber Broccoli Snap peas 8 oz radishes **Fruits:** 1 medium apple 1 pear 1 mango 8 oz frozen mango 4 oz frozen pineapple 8 oz fresh pineapple chunks 1 orange 1 lime 2 lemons Fresh berries of your choice 8 oz watermelon slices (if in season) **Herbs and Aromatics:** Basil leaves (approx. 2 cups) Fresh parsley Fresh dill Fresh cilantro Fresh thyme or rosemary (optional) 1 garlic bulb (approximately 8 cloves) Fresh ginger root (1 inch)	**Meat, Fish, and Other Proteins:** 4 chicken breasts (6 oz each) 1 lb ground turkey 2 cod fillets (6 oz each) 4 salmon fillets (5-6 oz each) 2 oz smoked salmon 1 can (5 oz) tuna ½ block firm tofu **Grains, Legumes, Nuts, and Seeds:** Quinoa Brown rice 2 cans (15 oz) chickpeas 1 can (15 oz) black beans Lentils Walnuts Almonds Mixed nuts Flaxseed Raw pumpkin seeds Chia seeds Almond butter Tahini **Eggs, Dairy, and Alternatives:** Eggs 8 oz full-fat Greek yogurt (2% if preferred) 8 oz coconut milk **Oils:** Extra Virgin Olive Oil **Other:** 8 small corn tortillas 1 loaf whole-grain bread 1 whole-grain wrap or tortilla 1 small container of capers Squares of dark chocolate (70% or higher) 1 small package shredded coconut (unsweetened) Honey
Anti-inflammatory Spice Mix Ingredients:	
ground turmeric ground cumin ground coriander paprika (regular or smoked) ground ginger garlic powder	onion powder ground cinnamon ground black pepper cayenne pepper (optional, for a bit of heat) thyme or oregano (optional)

Meal Plan - Week 2: Staying Determined

Day	Meal	Recipe Name
Day 8	**Breakfast**	Buckwheat Pancakes with Almond Butter and Banana Slices
	Snack 1	Sliced Pear Sprinkled with Cinnamon and Walnuts
	Lunch	Eggplant and Zucchini Gratin
	Snack 2	Roasted, Spiced Chickpeas
	Dinner	Spicy Beef and Veggie Stir-Fry
Day 9	**Breakfast**	Smoothie Bowl with Acai, Spinach, and Granola
	Snack 1	Sliced Bell Peppers with Guacamole
	Lunch	Rainbow Veggie Buddha Bowl
	Snack 2	Fresh Pineapple Sprinkled with Coconut Flakes
	Dinner	Grilled Salmon with Asparagus and Turmeric-Spiced Quinoa
Day 10	**Breakfast**	Turmeric Scrambled Eggs, Sautéed Kale, and Cherry Tomatoes
	Snack 1	Fresh Cucumber and Carrot Sticks with Tahini Dip
	Lunch	Spinach and Quinoa Salad with Pomegranate and Pecans
	Snack 2	Sliced Mango Sprinkled with Lime Juice and Chia Seeds
	Dinner	Chicken and Vegetable Skewers with Brown Rice and Tzatziki
Day 11	**Breakfast**	Berry Chia Seed Pudding with Almonds
	Snack 1	Brazil Nuts and Dark Chocolate Chips
	Lunch	Hummus, Veggie, and Quinoa Wrap
	Snack 2	Coconut Yogurt with Blueberries
	Dinner	Baked Eggplant Parmesan with Mixed Greens Salad
Day 12	**Breakfast**	Oatmeal with Cooked Apples, Flaxseeds, and Almond Butter
	Snack 1	Sliced Apple with Pumpkin Seeds and Cinnamon
	Lunch	Spinach and Lentil Salad with Pomegranate Seeds
	Snack 2	Hard-Boiled Egg with Cherry Tomatoes
	Dinner	Spiced Chicken with Roasted Cauliflower and Carrot Fries
Day 13	**Breakfast**	Smoothie Bowl with Spinach, Kiwi, Banana, and Granola
	Snack 1	Fresh Orange Slices with Almonds
	Lunch	Curried Chickpea and Sweet Potato Stew
	Snack 2	Homemade Granola Bar
	Dinner	Shrimp Stir-Fry with Broccoli, Snap Peas, and Brown Rice
Day 14	**Breakfast**	Buckwheat Groats with Berries, Chia Seeds, and Maple Syrup
	Snack 1	Fresh Strawberries with Dark Chocolate Dip
	Lunch	Quinoa Salad with Avocado, Spinach, and Cherry Tomatoes
	Snack 2	Celery Sticks Topped with Peanut Butter and Raisins
	Dinner	Pesto Chicken with Roasted Asparagus

Shopping List - Week 2

Produce:	**Proteins, Refrigerator, and Pantry:**
Leafy Greens:	**Meat, Fish, and Other Proteins:**
16 oz fresh spinach	2 chicken breasts (6 oz each)
16 oz mixed greens	8–10 medium shrimp
8 oz kale	4 oz lean beef
4 oz red cabbage, shredded	2 salmon fillets (6 oz each)
Vegetables:	½ block firm tofu
1 medium eggplant	**Grains, Legumes, Nuts, and Seeds:**
2 medium zucchinis	4 oz buckwheat flour
2 bell peppers	16 oz rolled oats
1 cucumber	1 can (15 oz) chickpeas
4 medium carrots	Brazil nuts
8 oz broccoli florets	**Eggs, Dairy, and Alternatives:**
8 oz snap peas	8 oz full-fat Greek yogurt (or 2%)
4 oz cherry tomatoes	2 oz grated Parmesan cheese (optional)
1 small tomato	4 oz coconut milk
8 oz asparagus	4 oz coconut yogurt
8 oz cauliflower florets	3 eggs
Fruits:	**Oils:**
1 banana	Sesame Oil (optional)
1 kiwi	**Other:**
2 pears	2 frozen acai berry smoothie packets
1 orange	8 oz vegetable broth
1 apple	Maple syrup (optional substitute for honey)
1 mango	Baking powder
8 oz fresh pineapple chunks	2 oz dried cranberries or raisins (unsweetened)
8 oz fresh blueberries	1 package dark chocolate chips
8 oz strawberries	
Other fresh berries of your choosing	
2 oz dried apricots	
Herbs and Aromatics:	
Fresh basil (approx. 2 cups for pesto)	
Fresh parsley	
Fresh dill	
Fresh cilantro	
1 small red onion	
1 small yellow or white onion	
1 garlic bulb (approx. 8 cloves)	
Fresh ginger root (1 inch)	

Pantry Items (Duplicates from Week 1)		
Quinoa	Almonds	Tahini
Brown Rice	Flaxseeds	Almond Butter
Lentils	Pumpkin Seeds	Extra Virgin Olive Oil
Walnuts	Chia Seeds	Honey

Meal Plan - Week 3: Hitting Your Stride

Day	Meal	Recipe Name
Day 15	**Breakfast**	Avocado Toast with Hemp Seeds, Arugula, and Poached Egg
	Snack 1	Fresh Grapefruit Topped with Honey and Mint
	Lunch	Kale and Sweet Potato Soup
	Snack 2	Baked Sweet Potato Chips
	Dinner	Honey-Ginger Salmon with Steamed Broccoli
Day 16	**Breakfast**	Warm Quinoa Porridge with Almond Milk, Pecans, & Peaches
	Snack 1	Sliced Cucumber with Olive Tapenade
	Lunch	Spinach and Strawberry Salad
	Snack 2	Celery Sticks Topped with Cashew Butter and Dates
	Dinner	Rosemary and Garlic Pork Chops with Mashed Cauliflower
Day 17	**Breakfast**	Sweet Potato and Spinach Hash with Poached Egg
	Snack 1	Fresh Apricots with Almonds
	Lunch	Lentil and Sweet Potato Salad
	Snack 2	Cottage Cheese with Pineapple
	Dinner	Lemon Herb Grilled Chicken with Roasted Sweet Potatoes
Day 18	**Breakfast**	Coconut Yogurt with Papaya, Chia Seeds, and Pistachios
	Snack 1	Sliced Apple Topped with Hemp Seeds and Almond Butter
	Lunch	Smoked Salmon and Avocado Wrap
	Snack 2	Cantaloupe Slices Drizzled with Lime Juice
	Dinner	Coconut Curry Lentil Soup
Day 19	**Breakfast**	Savory Oatmeal with Mushrooms, Spinach, and Walnuts
	Snack 1	Roasted Pumpkin Seeds with Sea Salt
	Lunch	Mediterranean Chickpea Salad
	Snack 2	Fresh Raspberries with Dark Chocolate Chips
	Dinner	Stuffed Bell Peppers with Quinoa and Turkey
Day 20	**Breakfast**	Blueberry and Flaxseed Smoothie with Ginger
	Snack 1	Fresh Figs with Goat Cheese
	Lunch	Stuffed Bell Peppers
	Snack 2	Radish Slices with Guacamole
	Dinner	Roasted Cod with Lemon and Thyme
Day 21	**Breakfast**	Millet Porridge with Coconut Milk, Berries, and Almonds
	Snack 1	Fresh Blackberries with Greek Yogurt
	Lunch	Butternut Squash and Kale Salad with Tahini Dressing
	Snack 2	Sunflower Seeds and Dried Cranberries
	Dinner	Chili Lime Shrimp Tacos with Shredded Cabbage

Shopping List - Week 3

Produce:	**Proteins, Refrigerator, and Pantry:**
Leafy Greens:	**Meat, Fish, and Other Proteins:**
5 cups spinach	2 chicken breasts (6 oz each)
2 cups kale	2 pork chops (6 oz each)
2 cups mixed greens	1 lb ground turkey
1 cup arugula	2 salmon fillets (6 oz each)
1 cup shredded cabbage	2 cod fillets (6 oz each)
Vegetables:	1 cup shrimp
4 medium sweet potatoes	2 oz smoked salmon
3 medium zucchini	**Grains, Legumes, Nuts, and Seeds:**
1 medium onion	4 oz millet
2 red onions	4 small corn tortillas
1 butternut squash	1 whole-grain wrap
1 cup broccoli florets	Whole-grain bread
1 cup cauliflower florets	1 can (15 oz) chickpeas
4 oz mushrooms (sliced)	1 can (15 oz) black beans
5-6 bell peppers	1 can (15 oz) corn kernels
2 carrots	1 small package sunflower seeds
4 oz cherry tomatoes	1 small package pecans
Fruits:	Cashew butter
2 bananas	1 small package pistachios (chopped)
1 grapefruit	Hemp seeds
4 oz raspberries	**Eggs, Dairy, and Alternatives:**
4 oz blackberries	4 eggs
4 oz papaya	4 oz low-fat cottage cheese
8 oz fresh pineapple chunks	4 oz Greek yogurt (low-fat)
4 oz cantaloupe	4 oz sour cream or Greek yogurt
8 oz frozen blueberries	8 oz cream cheese (optional for wrap)
1 peach	4 oz goat cheese
3 fresh apricots	8 oz coconut yogurt
4 fresh figs	8 oz unsweetened almond milk
1 apple	8 oz coconut milk
Herbs and Aromatics:	**Oils:**
Fresh parsley	Coconut Oil (optional)
Fresh cilantro	**Other:**
Fresh thyme (or dried)	Balsamic vinegar
Fresh rosemary (or dried)	White vinegar (optional)
Fresh mint	Dijon mustard
2 bulbs garlic (approx. 10 cloves)	8 oz vegetable broth
Fresh ginger root (1 inch)	4 oz tomato sauce
2 green onions (for sauce)	Curry powder

Pantry Items (Duplicates from Weeks 1 and 2)		
Quinoa	Almonds	Tahini
Brown Rice	Maple syrup (optional)	Extra Virgin Olive Oil
Rolled Oats	Pumpkin Seeds	Almond Butter
Lentils	Flaxseeds	Honey
Walnuts	Chia Seeds	

Meal Plan - Week 4: Seeing the Benefits

Day	Meal	Recipe Name
Day 22	**Breakfast**	Amaranth Porridge with Pear, Cinnamon, and Walnuts
	Snack 1	Sliced Pear Topped with Ricotta and Walnuts
	Lunch	Cauliflower Rice Bowl with Tofu and Veggies
	Snack 2	Avocado on Whole-Grain Toast
	Dinner	Moroccan-Spiced Lamb Chops with Roasted Vegetables
Day 23	**Breakfast**	Overnight Oats with Chia Seeds, Blueberries, and Maple Syrup
	Snack 1	Roasted Beet Hummus with Cucumber Slices
	Lunch	Grilled Chicken and Quinoa Salad
	Snack 2	Fresh Pineapple Sprinkled with Chili Powder
	Dinner	Coconut Curry Chicken with Spinach and Brown Rice
Day 24	**Breakfast**	Green Smoothie (with Berries and Banana)
	Snack 1	Fresh Papaya Sprinkled with Lime Juice and Coconut Flakes
	Lunch	Turkey, Avocado, and Spinach Wrap
	Snack 2	Cherry Tomatoes Tossed with Balsamic Glaze and Basil
	Dinner	Lemon-Garlic Chicken with Roasted Vegetables
Day 25	**Breakfast**	Acai Bowl with Banana, Granola, Chia Seeds, & Fresh Berries
	Snack 1	Bell Pepper Strips with Guacamole
	Lunch	Roasted Beet and Arugula Salad with Goat Cheese
	Snack 2	Watermelon Tossed with Fresh Mint
	Dinner	Roasted Pork Tenderloin with Apple and Sweet Potato
Day 26	**Breakfast**	Turmeric and Cinnamon Millet Porridge with Apples & Pecans
	Snack 1	Sliced Kiwi with Hemp Seeds
	Lunch	Soba Noodle Salad with Edamame and Sesame Dressing
	Snack 2	Energy Ball with Dates, Oats, Flaxseeds, and Almond Butter
	Dinner	Lentil and Vegetable Stew with Kale
Day 27	**Breakfast**	Buckwheat Pancakes with Blueberries and Maple Syrup
	Snack 1	Sliced Apple with Almond Butter
	Lunch	Roasted Tomato and Red Pepper Soup
	Snack 2	Fresh Raspberries with Almonds
	Dinner	Baked Halibut with Broccoli and Lemon-Garlic Sauce
Day 28	**Breakfast**	Oatmeal with Pear, Almonds, and a Drizzle of Honey
	Snack 1	Fresh Figs with Almond Butter
	Lunch	Chicken and Avocado Lettuce Wraps
	Snack 2	Dark Chocolate and Brazil Nuts
	Dinner	Lemon-Tahini Chicken with Roasted Veggies

Shopping List - Week 4

Produce:	**Proteins, Refrigerator, and Pantry:**
Leafy Greens:	**Meat, Fish, and Other Proteins:**
2 cups kale	5 chicken breasts (6 oz each)
2 cups spinach	1 pork tenderloin (8 - 10 oz)
1 cup shredded lettuce or 6 large leaves	1 cooked turkey breast
2 cups arugula	2 lamb chops (6 oz each)
Mixed greens	2 halibut fillets (6 oz each)
Vegetables:	1 block firm tofu
3 medium sweet potatoes	**Grains, Legumes, Nuts, and Seeds:**
1 small onion	Amaranth
2 red bell peppers	4 oz soba noodles
2 large tomatoes	1 can (15 oz) chickpeas
6 medium carrots	4 oz shelled edamame
4 oz cauliflower rice	1 small package sesame seeds
8 oz broccoli florets	**Eggs, Dairy, and Alternatives:**
8 oz Brussels sprouts	Unsweetened almond milk
2 cucumbers	8 oz full-fat coconut milk
4 cloves garlic	2 eggs
3 medium beets	8 oz ricotta cheese
Fruits:	2 oz goat cheese
2 pears	**Other:**
2 apples	Balsamic glaze
1 kiwi	Vanilla extract
2 bananas	Soy sauce, low sodium (or tamari if gluten-free)
1 frozen acai berry smoothie packet	
8 oz fresh blueberries	
8 oz raspberries	
4 oz frozen berries	
8 oz fresh pineapple chunks	
1 papaya	
4 fresh figs	
8 oz diced watermelon (if in season)	
Herbs and Aromatics:	
Fresh parsley	
Fresh cilantro	
Fresh basil	
Fresh mint	
Fresh rosemary (or dried)	
Fresh ginger root (1 inch)	

Pantry Items (Duplicates from Weeks 1, 2, and 3)		
Quinoa	Brazil Nuts	Tahini
Brown Rice	Dark Chocolate Squares	Extra Virgin Olive Oil
Rolled Oats	Maple syrup (optional)	Coconut oil
Millet	Pumpkin Seeds	Sesame oil
Lentils	Flaxseeds	Almond Butter
Walnuts	Chia Seeds	Honey
Almonds	Buckwheat Flour	Dijon mustard

Moving Forward

As you begin this 28-day anti-inflammatory meal plan, you're making a practical commitment to improving your health through balanced, nutritious meals. Each recipe that follows is crafted to help reduce inflammation while providing the nutrients your body needs. This plan is designed to make healthy eating simple, approachable, and enjoyable. Remember to listen to your body, adjust as needed, and take each day one meal at a time. By incorporating these meals into your routine, you're building habits that support long-term health and well-being.

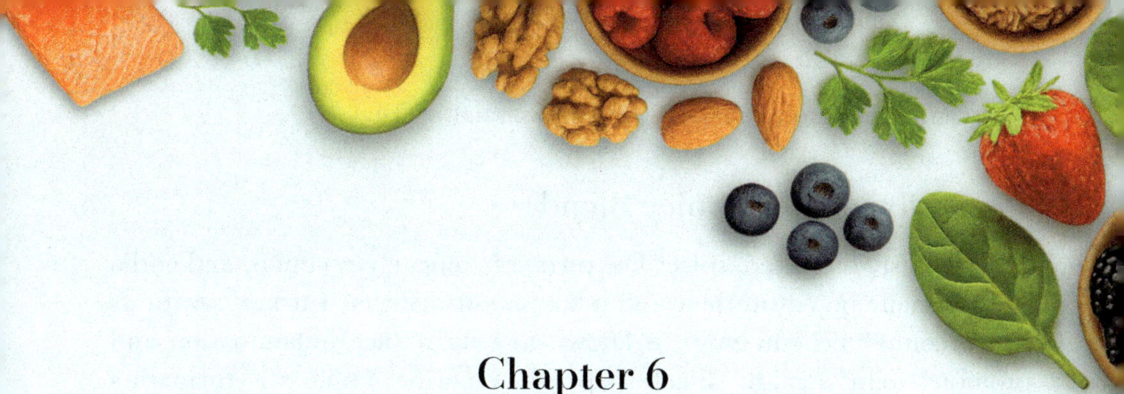

Chapter 6

Spices, Sauces, and Spreads

In the delicate dance of spices, sauces, and spreads lies the secret to elevating any meal into a nourishing experience. These vibrant additions not only awaken the senses but also carry potent anti-inflammatory benefits, weaving warmth and depth into every dish.

Anti-inflammatory spices, sauces, and spreads are essential elements in crafting delicious meals that support health goals. These additions provide depth of flavor while delivering a host of nutrients and compounds known to reduce inflammation. From the bold heat of turmeric and ginger to the subtle sweetness of cinnamon, spices offer a range of tastes and health benefits that can transform a dish. When combined with sauces and spreads made from wholesome ingredients, these elements elevate meals, adding layers of flavor and nutrition without compromising health.

Anti-Inflammatory Spice Blend

As previously discussed, spices like turmeric, ginger, cinnamon, and garlic are especially potent in their anti-inflammatory effects. Turmeric, with its active compound curcumin, is known to help reduce inflammation and promote joint health. Black pepper's piperine enhances turmeric's absorption in the body. Ginger has powerful anti-inflammatory and antioxidant properties that aid in digestion and soothe sore muscles. Cinnamon helps regulate blood sugar levels, making it a perfect addition to breakfast dishes or baked goods. Garlic, with its sulfur-containing compounds, supports immune health and is a flavorful addition to nearly any savory dish. Incorporating these spices into everyday meals is a simple way to elevate flavor and boost anti-inflammatory properties.

This chapter includes a versatile recipe for an anti-inflammatory spice blend, a flavorful mix of spices known for their health-boosting, anti-inflammatory properties. This blend combines turmeric, ginger, cinnamon, black pepper, and other warming spices, each selected for its unique benefits. This blend is perfect for seasoning a range of proteins, including chicken, tofu, and fish, and also adds depth to roasted vegetables, soups, and grain bowls. You can easily adjust the proportions of each spice to suit your taste. Preparing a batch of this spice mix in advance allows you to add an anti-inflammatory boost to your meals throughout the week, saving time while enriching your dishes with a warm, aromatic flavor.

Flavorful Anti-inflammatory Sauces and Spreads

Anti-inflammatory sauces and spreads allow us to enjoy creamy textures and rich flavors without relying on processed ingredients or added sugars. For instance, a tahini-based dressing combines sesame's nutty flavor with healthy fats and antioxidants. Blending tahini with lemon, garlic, and a dash of olive oil creates a sauce perfect for salads, roasted vegetables, or grain bowls. Similarly, pesto made with fresh basil, olive oil, and walnuts provides a burst of flavor and omega-3s, which help fight inflammation. Other sauce bases, like avocado and yogurt (or plant-based yogurt alternatives), add creaminess while delivering nutrients that support gut health and provide satiating fats.

Ultimately, anti-inflammatory spices, sauces, and spreads are key to making nutritious and enjoyable meals. By incorporating various elements, we can cater to diverse palates and dietary needs while nourishing the body. These flavorful additions demonstrate that healthy eating doesn't need to be bland or restrictive; rather, it can be an exploration of tastes and textures that enhance the enjoyment of food while supporting health. In this way, every meal becomes an opportunity to create balance, combining flavor with function in a way that truly brings the anti-inflammatory diet to life.

Anti-inflammatory Spices, Sauces, and Spreads - Recipes

The following recipes will elevate your anti-inflammatory meals and enhance your satisfaction with this way of eating. I encourage you to experiment with different flavor combinations as you progress with this plan.

Anti-Inflammatory Spice Blend

INGREDIENTS

- 2 tbsp ground turmeric
- 1 tbsp ground cumin
- 1 tbsp ground coriander
- 1 tbsp paprika (regular or smoked for a deeper flavor)
- 1 tsp ground ginger
- 1 tsp garlic powder
- 1 tsp onion powder
- ½ tsp ground cinnamon
- ½ tsp ground black pepper (to enhance the absorption of curcumin from turmeric)
- ¼ tsp cayenne pepper (optional, for a bit of heat)
- 1 tsp dried thyme or oregano (optional for added depth)

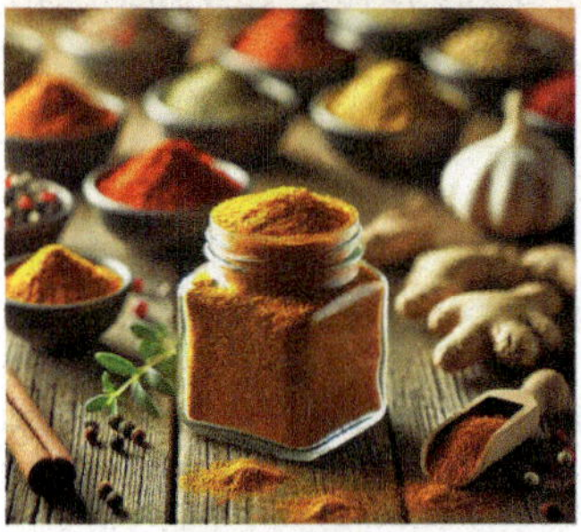

DIRECTIONS

1. Combine all the spices in a small bowl.
2. Transfer to an airtight container and store in a cool, dark place.

This versatile blend is perfect for seasoning chicken, tofu, and other proteins. It also adds a warm, aromatic flavor to roasted vegetables, soups, and grain bowls.

Roasted Red Pepper and Walnut Dip (Muhammara)

INGREDIENTS

- 2 large red bell peppers
- ½ cup walnuts
- 1 clove garlic, minced
- 2 tbsp olive oil
- 1 tbsp lemon juice
- 1 tsp cumin
- 1 tsp smoked paprika
- 1 tbsp pomegranate molasses (optional)
- Salt and pepper

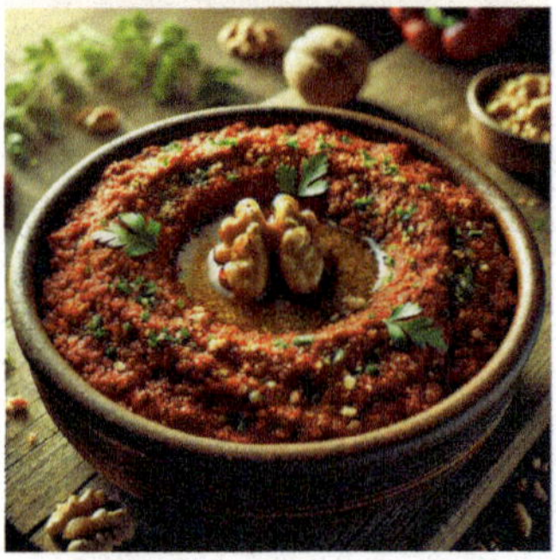

DIRECTIONS

1. Preheat oven to 400°F (200°C).
2. Roast whole peppers for 25-30 minutes until charred and soft.
3. Cover with plastic wrap to steam for 10 minutes.
4. Peel off skins and remove seeds.
5. Toast walnuts in a dry skillet over medium heat for 3-5 minutes.
6. Blend all ingredients in a food processor, adding extra olive oil or water to reach desired consistency.
7. Add salt and pepper to taste.
8. Drizzle with olive oil before serving.

NUTRITION

- Calories (per 2 tbsp serving): 120
- Macros: 10g fat, 5g carbs, 2g protein

This satisfying dip has a blend of smoky, nutty, and tangy flavors, perfect for pairing with vegetables or whole-grain crackers.

Tzatziki Sauce/Dip

DIRECTIONS

1. Grate cucumber and squeeze in a clean towel to remove excess water.
2. Mix all ingredients in a medium bowl.
3. Cover and refrigerate at least 30 minutes.
4. Serve with fresh vegetables, whole-grain pita bread, or crackers.
5. Use as a sauce for grilled chicken, tofu, or fish.
6. Add to grain bowls, wraps, or salads for extra creaminess and flavor.

INGREDIENTS

- 1 cup Greek yogurt
- 1 cucumber, grated
- 1 carrot, grated
- 2 cloves garlic, minced
- 1 tbsp olive oil
- 1 tbsp lemon juice
- 1 tbsp fresh dill, chopped
- ½ tsp salt
- ¼ tsp black pepper

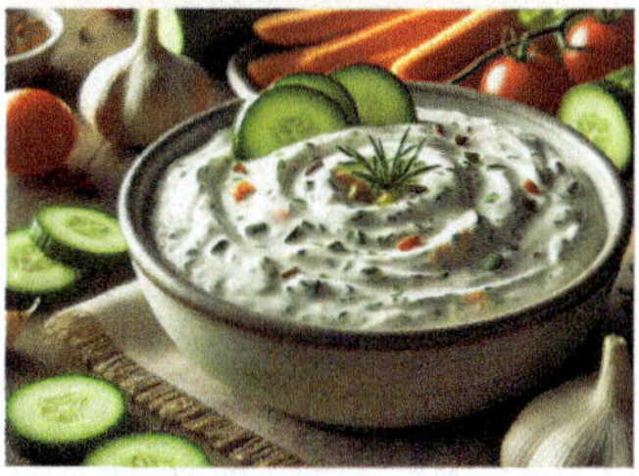

NUTRITION

- Calories (per 2 tbsp serving): 34
- Macros: 3g fat, 1g carbs, 2g protein

This refreshing, healthy sauce is packed with anti-inflammatory ingredients and perfect for a variety of dishes.

Guacamole Dip

DIRECTIONS

1. Seed and finely chop jalapeño, dice onion and tomato, and mince garlic
2. Mash pitted avocados with a fork until smooth but still slightly chunky.
3. Combine all ingredients.
4. Serve with vegetable sticks, whole-grain tortilla chips, or pita wedges.
5. Use to top tacos, burrito bowls, or grilled meats and tofu.
6. Spread on whole-grain toast or wraps for a quick snack or meal.

INGREDIENTS

- 3 ripe avocados
- 1 small red onion
- 1 small tomato
- 2 cloves garlic
- 1 jalapeño (optional for heat)
- ¼ cup fresh cilantro, chopped
- Juice of 1 lime
- ½ tsp cumin
- Salt and pepper, to taste

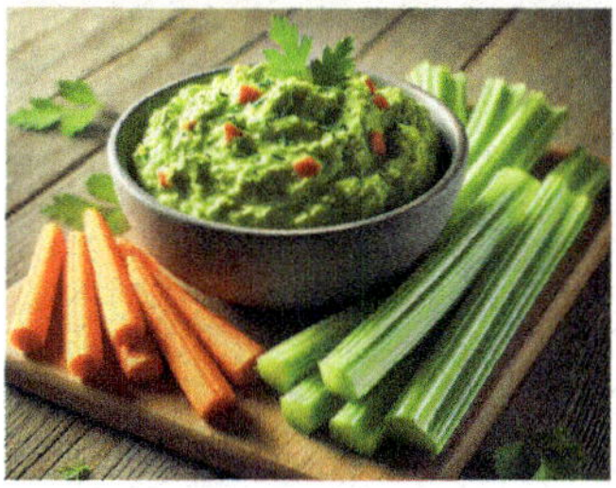

NUTRITION

- Calories (per 2 tbsp serving): 95
- Macros: 8g fat, 6g carbs, 1g protein

This classic and easy guacamole recipe is perfect as a dip, spread, or topping for your favorite anti-inflammatory meals.

Classic Hummus

INGREDIENTS

- 1 can (15 oz) chickpeas
- ¼ cup tahini
- 2-3 tbsp olive oil, plus extra for drizzling
- 1-2 cloves garlic, minced
- Juice of 1 lemon
- ½ tsp ground cumin
- ½ tsp salt
- Paprika, for garnish (optional)

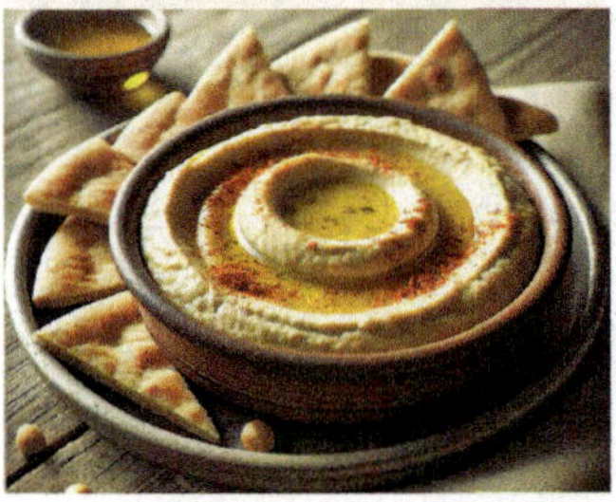

DIRECTIONS

1. Drain and rinse chickpeas, reserving a few tablespoons of liquid.
2. Combine the first 7 ingredients in a food processor. Blend until smooth.
3. Add reserved chickpea liquid, one tbsp at a time to reach desired consistency.
4. Top with olive oil and paprika.
5. Serve with fresh vegetables, whole-grain pita, or crackers. Use as a spread for sandwiches, wraps, or burgers, or add a dollop to salads or grain bowls for added creaminess and flavor.

NUTRITION

- Calories (per 2 tbsp serving): 90
- Macros: 7g fat, 6g carbs, 2g protein

This classic hummus recipe is packed with anti-inflammatory ingredients like garlic, olive oil, and tahini.

Roasted Beet Hummus

INGREDIENTS

- 1 small beet, roasted and peeled
- 1 cup chickpeas, rinsed and drained
- 1 tbsp tahini
- 1 garlic clove
- Juice of 1 lemon
- 1 tbsp olive oil
- Salt and pepper to taste

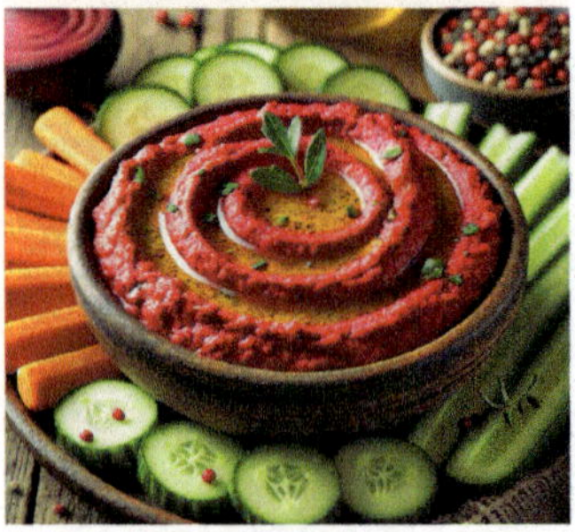

DIRECTIONS

1. Preheat oven to 400°F (200°C).
2. Wrap beet in foil and roast for 45-60 minutes, or until tender.
3. Allow beet to cool, then peel.
4. Combine all ingredients in a food processor and blend until smooth and creamy. Add more water or olive oil to reach desired consistency.
5. Drizzle with olive oil prior to serving.

NUTRITION

- Calories (per 2 tbsp serving): 60
- Macros: 3g fat, 6g carbs, 25g protein

This hummus recipe adds a burst of color and flavor to your snack or meal, in addition to its anti-inflammatory benefits.

Olive Tapenade

DIRECTIONS

1. Add olives, capers, garlic, parsley, and lemon juice to a food processor.
2. Pulse until coarsely chopped.
3. Drizzle olive oil into food processor until just combined.
4. Add salt and pepper to taste (Be careful not to over-salt as olives and capers are already salty).

INGREDIENTS

- 1 cup pitted Kalamata olives (or a mix of green and black olives, if preferred)
- 2 tbsp capers, drained
- 2 cloves garlic, minced
- 2 tbsp fresh parsley, chopped

NUTRITION

- Calories (per tblsp): 50
- Macros: 5g fat, 1g carbs, 0g protein

This flavorful, quick, and savory spread is perfect for pairing with whole wheat crackers, bread, or as a topping for grilled vegetables and proteins.

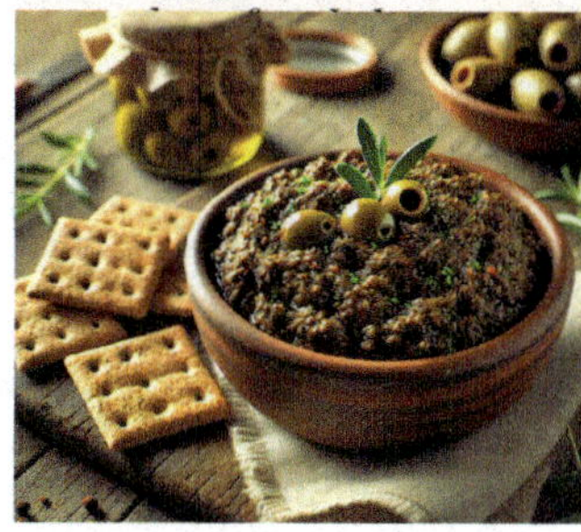

Cilantro Lime Sauce

DIRECTIONS

1. Add all ingredients to a blender or food processor and pulse until mixture reaches the desired consistency.
2. Serve with almost any dish.
3. Store in an airtight container in the refrigerator for up to 1 week.
4. Stir before serving.

INGREDIENTS

- 2 tbsp olive oil
- ½ avocado (peeled and pitted)
- ¼ cup water
- ½ cup chopped green onion
- ¾ cup cilantro leaves
- 2 cloves garlic, minced
- Juice of 1 lime
- ½ teaspoon salt
- ½ cup greek yogurt

NUTRITION

- Calories (per serving, approx. 2 tbsp): 60
- Macros: 6g fat, 2g carbs, 1g protein

This refreshing cilantro lime sauce is ideal as a dressing, marinade, or drizzle over tacos and roasted veggies.

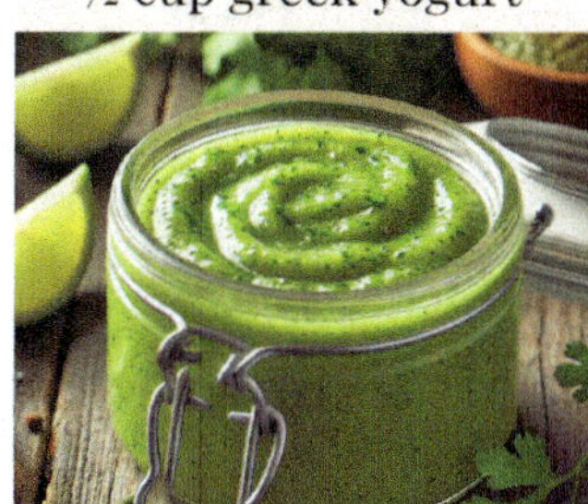

Lemon Tahini Dressing

INGREDIENTS

- 2 tbsp tahini
- 2 tbsp olive oil
- 2 tbsp lemon juice
- 2 tsp honey
- 2 cloves garlic, minced
- Salt and pepper to taste

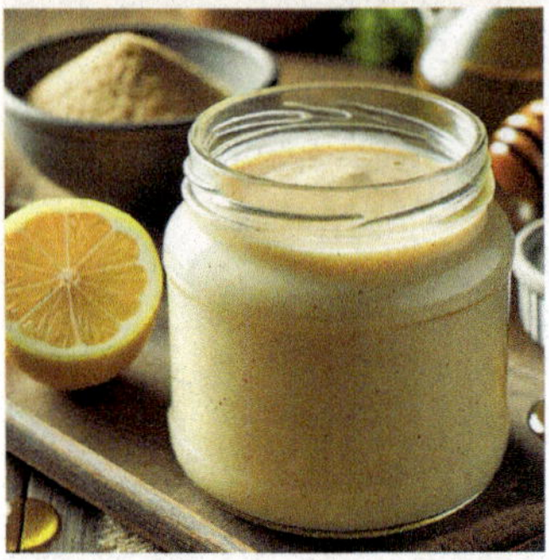

DIRECTIONS

1. In a small bowl, whisk together the tahini, olive oil, lemon juice, honey, minced garlic, salt, and pepper.
2. Transfer to a sealable container.
3. Can be stored in the refrigerator for up to 7 days in an airtight container.
4. Stir before each use.

NUTRITION

- Calories (per tblsp): 48
- Macros: 4g fat, 2g carbs, 1g protein

This creamy dressing is great for salads, grain bowls, and roasted vegetables with the added benefit of healthy fats.

Balsamic Vinaigrette

INGREDIENTS

- ¼ cup balsamic vinegar
- ¾ cup extra-virgin olive oil
- 1 clove garlic, minced
- 1 tsp Dijon mustard
- 1 tsp honey or maple syrup (optional, for a touch of sweetness)
- Salt and pepper to taste

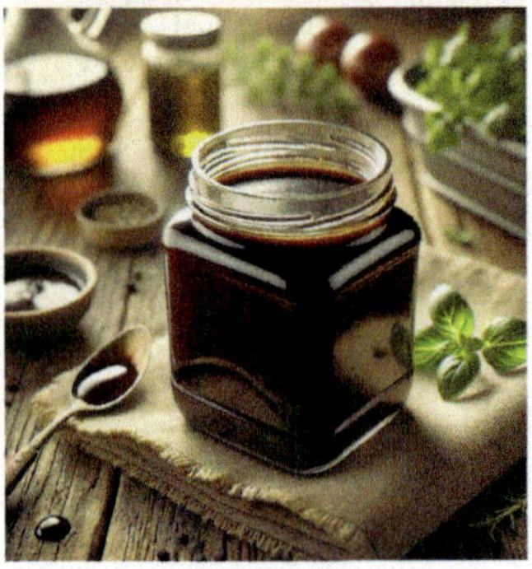

DIRECTIONS

1. In a small bowl or jar, whisk together the balsamic vinegar, garlic, Dijon mustard, honey or maple syrup, salt, and pepper.
2. Gradually whisk in the olive oil until the dressing is emulsified. Alternatively, you can combine all ingredients in a jar, secure the lid, and shake well to mix.
3. Taste the dressing and adjust seasoning and sweetener if needed.
4. Store in an airtight container in the refrigerator for up to 1 week. Shake well before using.

NUTRITION

- Calories (per tblsp): 80
- Macros: 8g fat, 1g carbs, 0g protein

This simple and tangy balsamic vinaigrette is perfect for salads, roasted vegetables, or as a marinade.

Lemon Herb Dressing

DIRECTIONS

1. Place olive oil, lemon juice, Dijon mustard, garlic, parsley, and basil or thyme in a small jar with lid.
2. Add salt and pepper to taste.
3. Secure the lid and shake until well combined.
4. Drizzle over salads, vegetables, or grain dishes.
5. Stir or shake well before each use, as separation may occur.

INGREDIENTS

- ¼ cup olive oil
- 2 tbsp fresh lemon juice
- 1 tsp Dijon mustard
- 1 clove garlic, minced
- 1 tbsp fresh parsley, chopped
- 1 tbsp fresh basil or thyme, chopped
- Salt and pepper

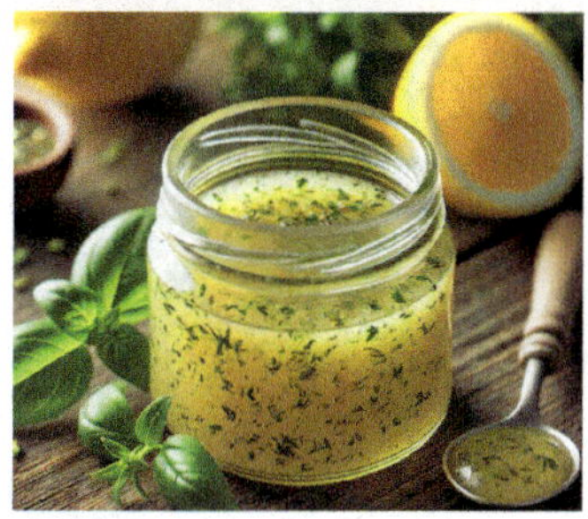

NUTRITION

- Calories (per tbsp): 60
- Macros: 6g fat, 1g carbs, 0g protein

This fresh and tangy lemon herb dressing is a versatile addition to salads, roasted vegetables, or grain bowls.

Creamy Mango Dressing

DIRECTIONS

1. Blend mango cubes, olive oil, lime juice, garlic, ginger, salt, honey, and water in a blender, until smooth and creamy.
2. Transfer to a bowl and stir in finely chopped habanero and cilantro. Adjust to taste.
3. Pour into an airtight glass jar and refrigerate until ready to use.

INGREDIENTS

- 1 cup ripe mango, cubed
- ¼ cup olive oil
- 3-4 tbsp lime juice
- 1 clove garlic
- 1 tsp grated ginger
- 1 tsp salt
- 1 tbsp honey
- ¼ cup water
- 1 habanero pepper
- 1 stalk fresh cilantro

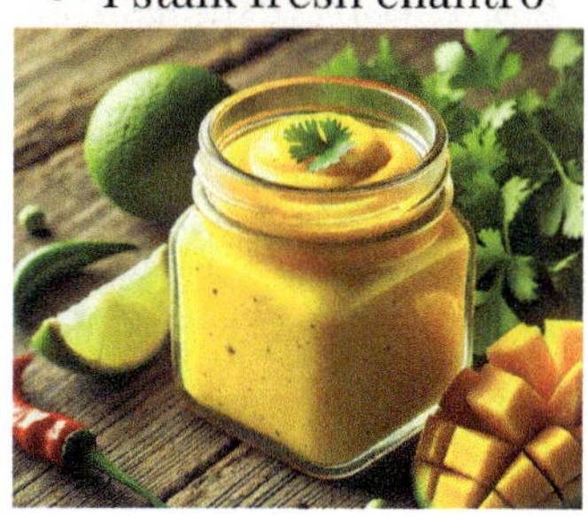

NUTRITION

- Calories (per 2 tbsp): 50
- Macros: 4g fat, 4g carbs, 0g protein

This vibrant mango dressing, inspired by Caribbean flavors, is great as a dressing, dip or a sauce.

Basil Walnut Pesto

INGREDIENTS

- 2 cups fresh basil
- ¼ cup walnuts
- 2 cloves garlic
- ¼ cup olive oil
- 2 tbsp lemon juice
- ¼ cup grated Parmesan cheese (or nutritional yeast for a dairy-free option)
- Salt and pepper

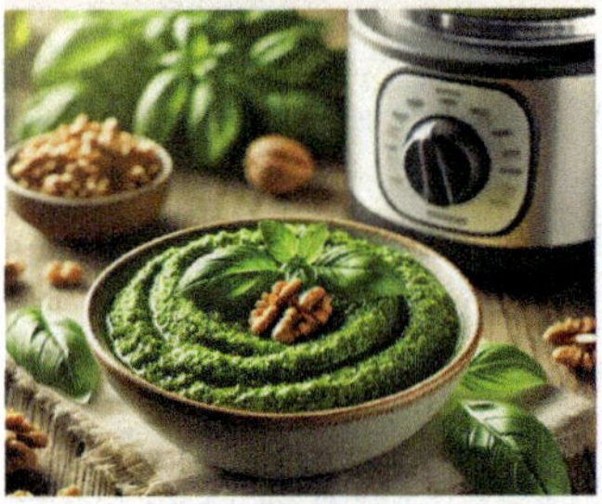

DIRECTIONS

1. Combine basil leaves, walnuts, minced garlic, lemon juice, and Parmesan cheese (or nutritional yeast) in a food processor. Pulse until the mixture is finely chopped.
2. With the food processor running, slowly drizzle in the olive oil until the pesto becomes smooth and creamy.
3. Season with salt and pepper to taste.

NUTRITION

- Calories (per tbsp): 100
- Macros: 10g fat, 1g carbs, 2g protein

This basil walnut pesto is rich in healthy fats and pairs well with pasta, zucchini noodles, or as a spread for sandwiches.

Homemade Marinara Sauce

INGREDIENTS

- 1 tbsp olive oil
- 1 small onion
- 1 large carrot
- 3 cloves garlic
- 1 tsp dried oregano
- 1 tsp dried basil
- ½ tsp ground turmeric
- 28 oz can crushed tomatoes
- Salt and pepper
- 1-2 tbsp fresh basil

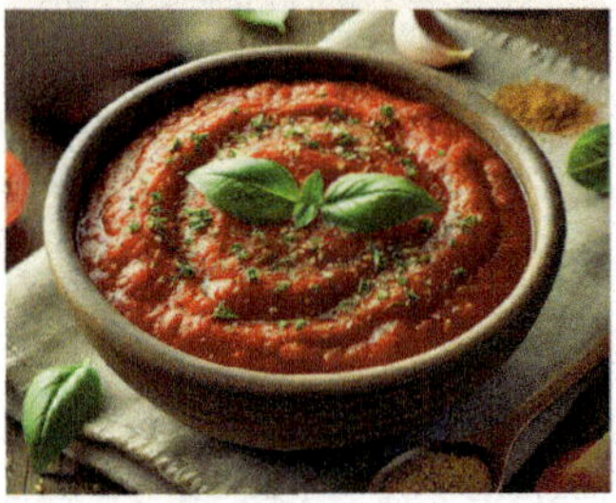

DIRECTIONS

1. Sauté finely chopped onion and grated carrot in olive oil for about 5 minutes until softened.
2. Add minced garlic, oregano, dried basil, and turmeric.
3. Sauté for 1-2 minutes until fragrant.
4. Stir in crushed tomatoes.
5. Season with salt and pepper to taste.
6. Reduce heat to low, cover and simmer 20-25 minutes, stirring occasionally.
7. Stir in chopped fresh basil before serving.

NUTRITION

- Calories (per ½ cup serving): 70
- Macros: 3g fat, 9g carbs, 2g protein

This sauce is a wholesome addition to pasta and veggies or as a base for other dishes.

Your Review Can Make a Difference

"Health is a journey, not a destination, and every step forward is a step toward a brighter tomorrow."

— Wellness Adage

Isn't it incredible how one choice, one moment, or one piece of advice can spark lasting change in someone's life? As you take steps to calm your inflammation and embrace a healthier lifestyle, please consider helping me reach others who need this information.

Your experiences and insights are powerful, and leaving a review for *Calm Your Inflammation Anti-inflammatory Diet* could be the encouragement someone else needs to start their path to better health. Your review may inspire someone who might be struggling to find answers. Your words could provide hope and guidance for:

• A parent longing for the energy to enjoy precious moments with their children.

• A grandparent seeking relief to fully embrace their time with family.

• A friend searching for effective solutions to feel better and live better.

It's a small gesture with a big impact and it only takes a moment.

You can pop over to Amazon with this link:

https://www.amazon.com/review/review-your-purchases/?asin=1963554035

Or scan this QR code with the camera on your phone and touch the link that pops up. The rest is even easier! Just follow the prompts to leave your review. It takes less than 60 seconds!

Thank you for being part of this shared mission to build healthier, stronger lives. Together, through learning, sharing, and supporting each other, we can make a meaningful difference.

Warmest Regards,
Brenda

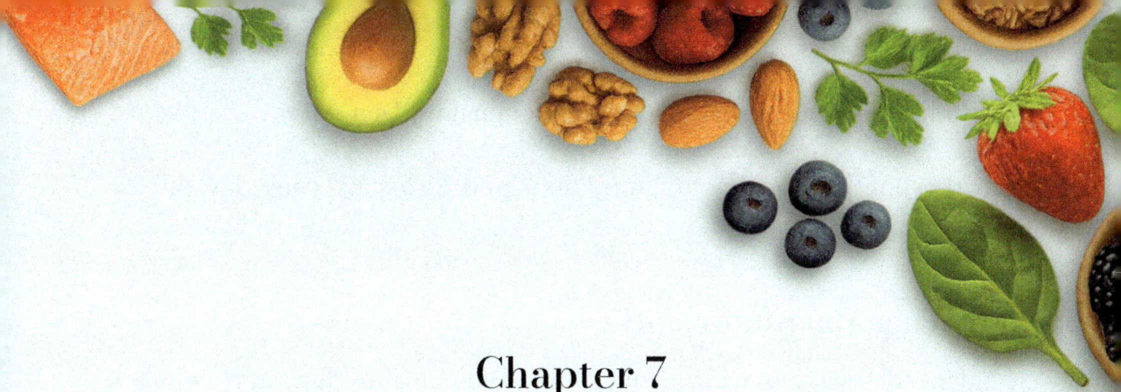

Chapter 7

Great Start Breakfasts

In the stillness of morning, when the world whispers and daylight creeps through the curtains, the initial act of nourishment sets the tone for the day. It is here, in this dawn-lit space, that the foundation for anti-inflammatory eating begins, one meal at a time.

Breakfast represents our first choice for how we will begin our day. It should provide the essential nutrients and energy needed to fuel both body and mind. In an anti-inflammatory diet, the first meal of the day takes on even greater importance, as it's a prime opportunity to incorporate ingredients that help reduce inflammation, support gut health, and stabilize blood sugar levels.

A well-balanced, anti-inflammatory breakfast helps curb mid-morning cravings. It promotes sustained energy and mental clarity, setting you up for success from the very start. This chapter explores a variety of breakfast options that are quick, delicious, and packed with anti-inflammatory ingredients—like berries, leafy greens, whole grains, healthy fats, and spices. Whether you're looking for a quick smoothie, a hearty bowl of oatmeal, or a savory breakfast scramble, these recipes are designed to nourish your body, calm inflammation, and kick-start your day on the right foot.

Balancing Macronutrients

A balanced breakfast with a mix of proteins, healthy fats, and complex carbohydrates is vital to maintaining energy and reducing inflammation. Incorporating protein-rich foods such as eggs, Greek yogurt, or plant-based options like chia seeds, quinoa, and nuts into your breakfast provides the nutrients needed to fuel the morning. A protein-packed breakfast will satisfy your appetite and set the stage for mindful eating throughout the day, helping you make balanced, intentional food choices.

Healthy fats, particularly those rich in omega-3s like flaxseeds and walnuts, help calm inflammation and support overall health. Choosing complex carbohydrates, such as fiber-rich fruits, vegetables, and whole grains, will provide a steady source of energy without the sharp blood sugar spikes caused by refined carbohydrate options. This balanced approach ensures each macronutrient works together to fuel your morning, promoting a day of sustained energy.

Quick Breakfast Ideas and On-the-Go Options

Creating quick and nourishing breakfasts doesn't have to be a challenge, even on the busiest of mornings. A simple smoothie made with leafy greens, hemp seeds, and a handful of berries packs a powerful punch of antioxidants, protein, and healthy fats in just minutes. Avocado toast on sprouted grain bread, topped with a sprinkle of seeds, offers a satisfying start that's both delicious and full of nutrients. These breakfasts come together in under 15 minutes, proving that starting the day with a healthy meal is achievable and a flavorful way to set a positive tone for the hours ahead.

For mornings when time is tight, grab-and-go breakfasts can be lifesavers. Overnight oats, prepared the night before with almond milk, cinnamon, and fresh blueberries, are a quick, ready-to-eat option that combines convenience with balanced nutrition. Simple, make-ahead meals provide the nourishment you need without sacrificing precious time, ensuring that even the busiest mornings are met with a nutritious start.

Avoiding added sugars doesn't mean sacrificing flavor at breakfast. Chia pudding, soaked overnight in coconut milk with a touch of vanilla and naturally sweetened with mashed banana, offers a satisfying, low-sugar alternative that feels indulgent yet balanced. Sweetening recipes with natural sugars like pure maple syrup or honey can satisfy your sweet tooth without promoting inflammation. Low-sugar options fuel the body with whole foods, providing steady energy without the highs and lows of sugary breakfasts.

Anti-Inflammatory Breakfast Recipes

The breakfasts in this chapter are more than just recipes—they are invitations to start each day with intention and care. By choosing ingredients that support your health, you can create morning meals that are quick and easy but also deeply nourishing.

Whether blending a smoothie, prepping overnight oats, or cooking a family breakfast, each choice reflects a commitment to fueling your body and supporting your overall well-being. These recipes remind us that even the simplest of meals can have a lasting impact on our health, helping us step into the day feeling energized, balanced, and ready to take on whatever comes next.

Smoothie with Spinach, Pineapple, Ginger, and Flaxseed

INGREDIENTS

- 1 cup spinach
- ½ cup frozen pineapple
- 1 tsp fresh ginger, grated
- 1 tbsp flaxseed
- 1 cup almond milk

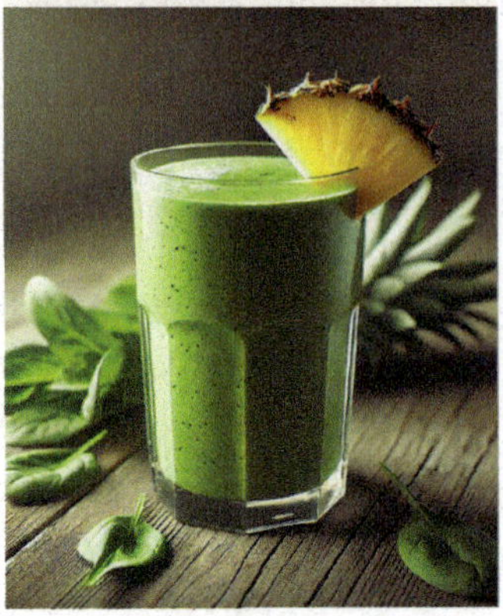

DIRECTIONS

1. Place all ingredients in a blender.
2. Blend all ingredients until smooth.
3. Serve immediately and enjoy!

NUTRITION

- Calories: 180
- Macros: 6g fat, 28g carbs, 4g protein

This smoothie is a refreshing and nutrient-rich blend that supports digestion and reduces inflammation, thanks to its anti-inflammatory ingredients like ginger and omega-3-rich flaxseed.

Chia Seed Pudding with Mango, Coconut Milk, and Pistachios

INGREDIENTS

- 3 tbsp chia seeds
- 1 cup coconut milk
- ½ cup mango, diced
- 2 tbsp pistachios, chopped

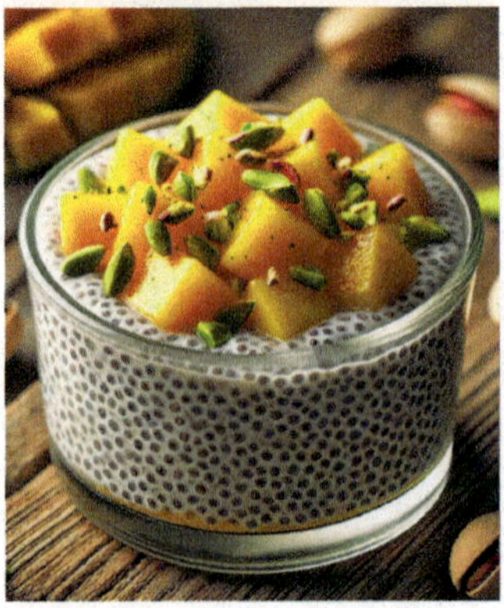

DIRECTIONS

1. Mix chia seeds and coconut milk.
2. Refrigerate overnight.
3. Top with diced mango and pistachios before serving.

NUTRITION

- Calories: 280
- Macros: 18g fat, 28g carbs, 6g protein

This creamy, nutrient-dense treat is rich in omega-3s, antioxidants, and anti-inflammatory properties, making it a delicious and wholesome option for a healthy snack or breakfast.

Smoked Salmon and Avocado Breakfast Bowl with Capers

DIRECTIONS

1. Arrange smoked salmon, sliced avocado, and mixed greens in a bowl.
2. Drizzle with olive oil and lemon juice.
3. Sprinkle with capers.

INGREDIENTS

- 2 oz smoked salmon
- ½ avocado, sliced
- 1 cup mixed greens
- 1 tbsp capers
- 1 tbsp olive oil
- Juice of ½ lemon

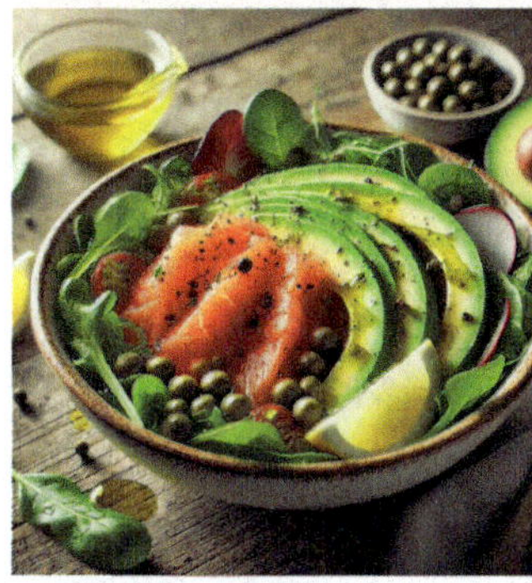

NUTRITION

- Calories: 350
- Macros: 28g fat, 12g carbs, 15g protein

Salmon is rich in omega-3 fatty acids, which have potent anti-inflammatory properties to help reduce inflammation and support heart and joint health.

Quinoa Breakfast Bowl with Coconut, Berries, and Almond Butter

DIRECTIONS

1. Cook quinoa as directed.
2. Place cooked quinoa in a bowl.
3. Top with mixed berries, shredded coconut, and almond butter. Drizzle with honey if desired.

INGREDIENTS

- 1 cup cooked quinoa
- ½ cup mixed berries (strawberries, blueberries, raspberries)
- 1 tbsp shredded coconut
- 1 tbsp almond butter
- 1 tsp honey (optional)

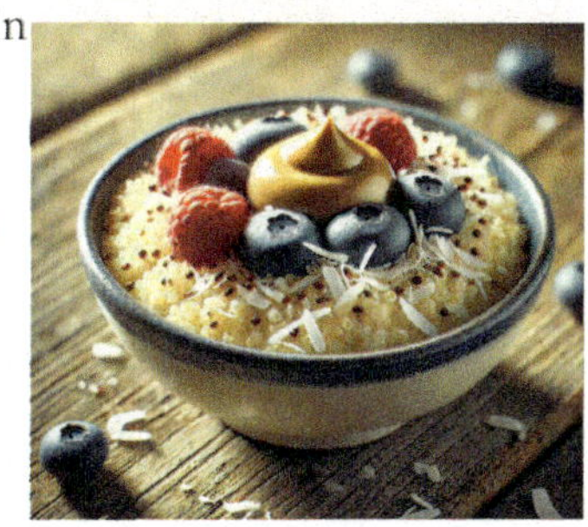

NUTRITION

- Calories: 320
- Macros: 14g fat, 45g carbs, 8g protein

Quinoa can be made ahead and reheated or served cold. Adding your favorite toppings elevates this delicious breakfast bowl.

Greek Yogurt Parfait with Strawberries and Walnuts

INGREDIENTS

- 1 cup Greek yogurt
- ¼ cup chopped walnuts
- ½ cup strawberries, sliced
- 1 tbsp chia seeds
- 1 tsp honey

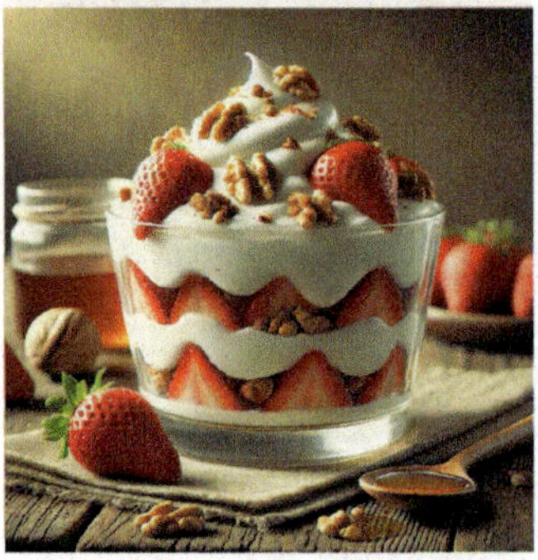

DIRECTIONS

1. Layer yogurt, strawberries, walnuts, and chia seeds in a glass bowl or dessert dish.
2. Repeat layers 2 to 3 times, depending on preference.
3. Drizzle with honey.

NUTRITION

- Calories: 320
- Macros: 18g fat, 28g carbs, 20g protein

This Greek Yogurt Parfait is packed with protein, healthy fats, and delicious flavors that make a perfect start to your day or a satisfying treat anytime!

Scrambled Eggs with Spinach, Tomatoes, and Avocado Toast

INGREDIENTS

- 2 eggs
- 1 cup spinach
- ½ cup cherry tomatoes, halved
- 1 tsp extra virgin olive oil
- 1 slice whole-grain bread, toasted
- ½ avocado, mashed

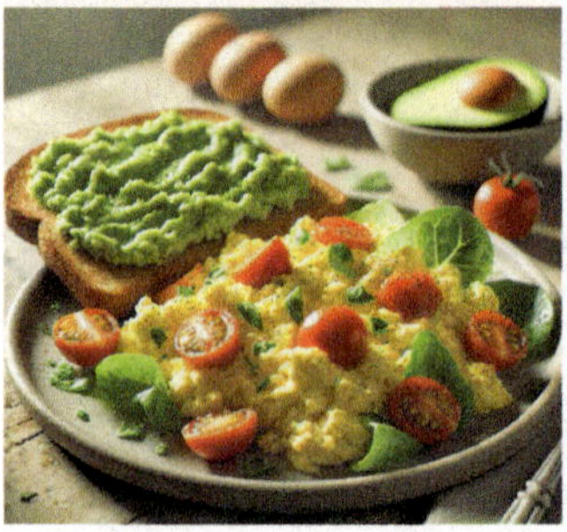

DIRECTIONS

1. Scramble eggs in extra virgin olive oil with spinach and tomatoes.
2. Spread mashed avocado on toast and serve with scrambled eggs.
3. Enjoy!

NUTRITION

- Calories: 320
- Macros: 18g fat, 28g carbs, 20g protein

This easy and delicious recipe combines creamy avocado toast with protein-packed eggs and fresh vegetables, to give you a satisfying start to your day!

Chia Seed Pudding with Coconut Milk and Mango

DIRECTIONS

1. Mix chia seeds and coconut milk.
2. Cover and refrigerate overnight or for at least 4 hours.
3. Top with mango chunks and shredded coconut before serving.

INGREDIENTS

- 3 tbsp chia seeds
- 1 cup coconut milk (or milk of choice)
- ½ cup fresh mango chunks
- 1 tbsp shredded coconut

NUTRITION

- Calories: 320
- Macros: 25g fat, 28g carbs, 5g protein

This make-ahead meal is perfect for busy mornings. You can substitute toppings of choice for personal taste and added variety

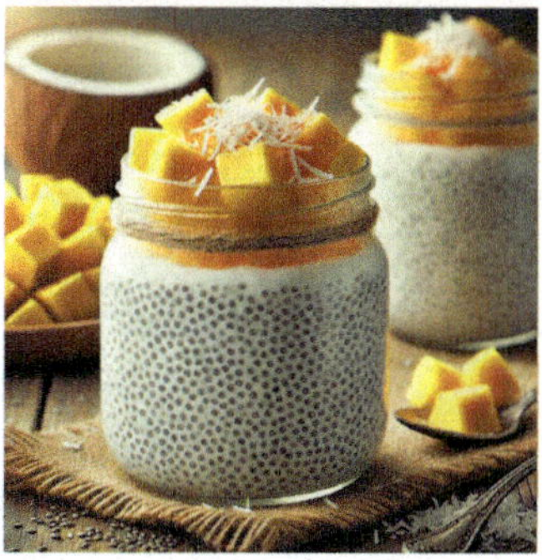

Buckwheat Pancakes with Almond Butter and Banana Slices

DIRECTIONS

1. Mix flour, egg, almond milk, and baking powder to form a batter.
2. Cook pancakes on a non-stick skillet.
3. Top with almond butter, banana slices, and chopped almonds, if desired.

INGREDIENTS

- ½ cup buckwheat flour
- 1 egg
- ½ cup almond milk
- 1 tsp baking powder
- 1 tbsp almond butter
- 1 banana, sliced
- Chopped almonds (optional)

NUTRITION

- Calories: 320
- Macros: 15g fat, 45g carbs, 10g protein

These pancakes can be made ahead and refrigerated or frozen, then reheated for a quick breakfast in the morning.

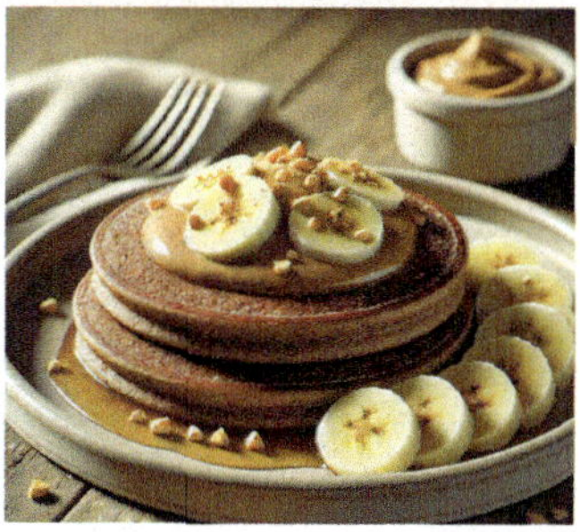

Smoothie Bowl with Acai, Spinach, and Granola

INGREDIENTS

- 1 frozen acai berry smoothie packet
- 1 cup spinach
- ½ cup almond milk
- 1 tbsp chia seeds
- ¼ cup granola
- Fresh berries for topping

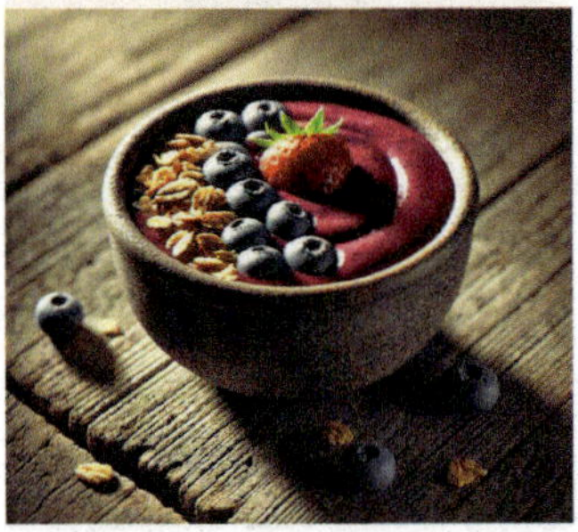

DIRECTIONS

1. Place acai, spinach, and almond milk in blender.
2. Blend until thick and smooth.
3. Top with chia seeds, granola, and berries.
4. Enjoy!

NUTRITION

- Calories: 350
- Macros: 15g fat, 55g carbs, 7g protein

This is a quick and easy choice for a nutritious start to your day. You can use whichever milk you choose and vary your toppings.

Turmeric Scrambled Eggs with Kale & Cherry Tomatoes

INGREDIENTS

- 2 eggs
- 1 cup kale, chopped
- ½ cup cherry tomatoes, halved
- 1 tsp turmeric
- 1 tbsp olive oil
- Salt and pepper to taste

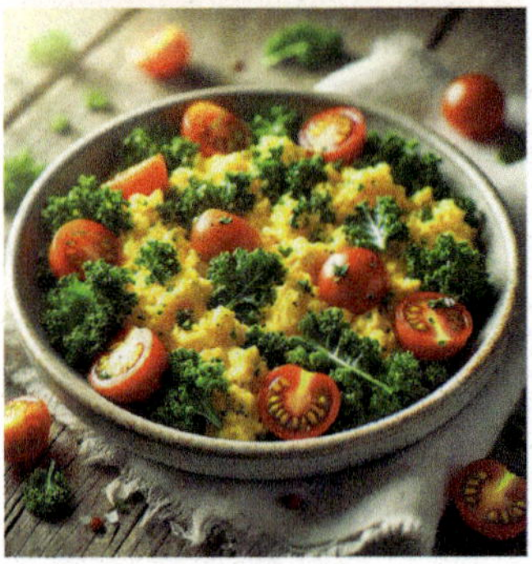

DIRECTIONS

1. Heat olive oil in a pan, add kale and cherry tomatoes, and sauté until softened.
2. Whisk eggs with turmeric, salt, and pepper, then pour into the pan.
3. Scramble until cooked through and serve.

NUTRITION

- Calories: 280
- Macros: 22g fat, 10g carbs, 14g protein

This delicious recipe combines protein-packed scrambled eggs and fresh vegetables, and the anti-inflammatory properties of Turmeric.

Berry Chia Seed Pudding with Almonds

INGREDIENTS

- 3 tbsp chia seeds
- 1 cup unsweetened almond milk
- ½ cup mixed berries (fresh or frozen)
- 1 tbsp sliced or whole almonds
- 1 tsp maple syrup

DIRECTIONS

1. Mix chia seeds and almond milk in a jar or bowl. Stir well, cover, and refrigerate overnight.
2. Top with mixed berries, almonds, and a drizzle of maple syrup before serving.

NUTRITION

- Calories: 300
- Macros: 18g fat, 32g carbs, 8g protein

This quick-start, anti-inflammatory breakfast is perfect for busy mornings!

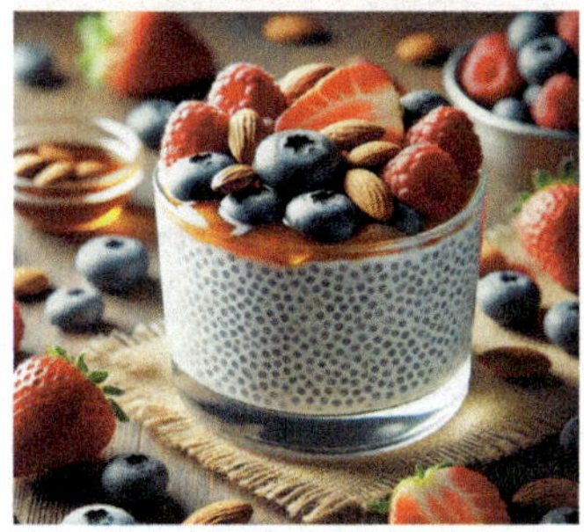

Oatmeal with Cooked Apples, Flaxseeds, and Almond Butter

INGREDIENTS

- ½ cup rolled oats
- 1 apple, diced
- 1 tsp cinnamon
- 1 tbsp flaxseeds
- 1 tbsp almond butter
- 1 cup water or almond milk

DIRECTIONS

1. In a saucepan, cook oats as directed, with water or almond milk.
2. In a separate pan, cook apples with a splash of water and cinnamon until soft.
3. Top oatmeal with apples, flaxseeds, and almond butter.

NUTRITION

- Calories: 250
- Macros: 6g fat, 48g carbs, 5g protein

This delicious, hearty breakfast is a great start to any morning.

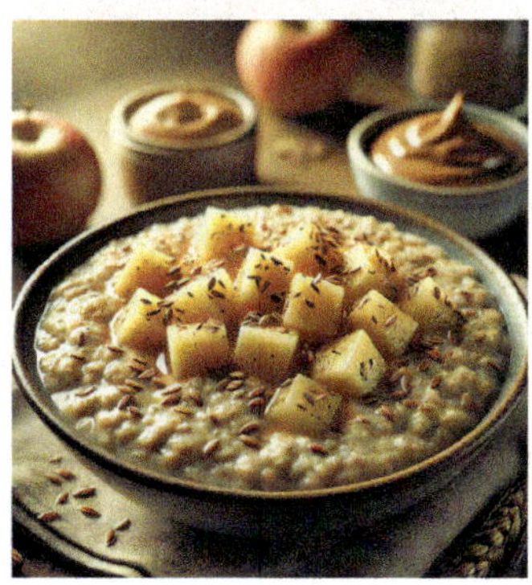

Smoothie Bowl with Spinach, Kiwi, Banana, and Granola

INGREDIENTS

- 1 cup fresh spinach
- 1 kiwi, peeled
- 1 banana
- ½ cup almond milk
- ¼ cup granola

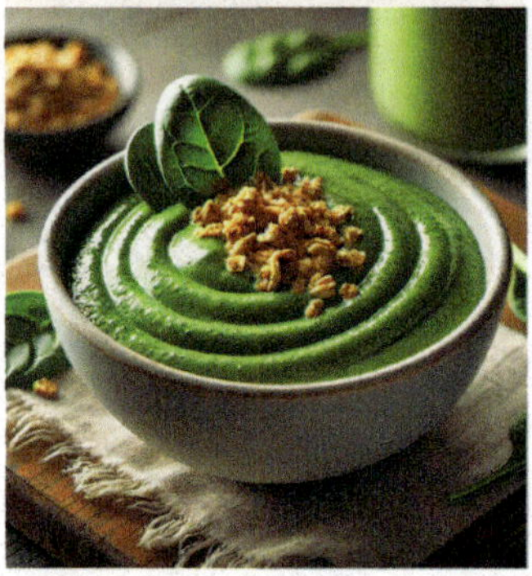

DIRECTIONS

1. Add spinach, kiwi, banana, and almond milk to a blender.
2. Blend until smooth.
3. Pour into a bowl.
4. Top with granola before serving.

NUTRITION

- Calories: 350
- Macros: 10g fat, 65g carbs, 7g protein

This is a quick and easy choice for a nutritious start to your day. You can use whichever milk you choose and vary your toppings.

Buckwheat Groats with Berries, Chia Seeds, and Maple Syrup

INGREDIENTS

- ½ cup buckwheat groats (hulled seeds of the buckwheat plant)
- 1 cup water
- ½ cup mixed berries
- 1 tbsp chia seeds
- 1 tsp maple syrup

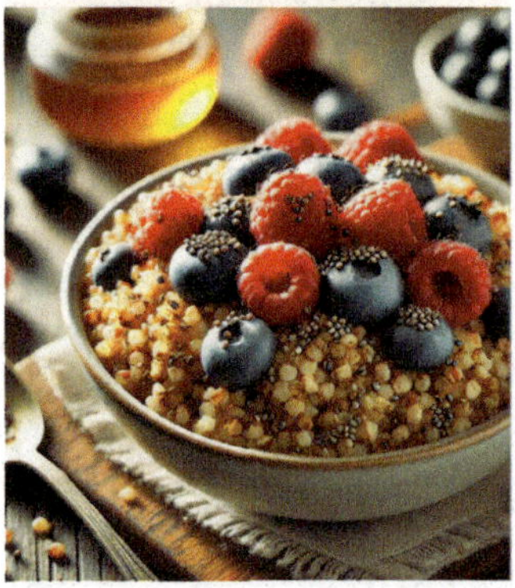

DIRECTIONS

1. Cook buckwheat groats in water over medium heat until tender, about 10 - 15 minutes.
2. Add to a bowl.
3. Top with berries, chia seeds, and maple syrup.

NUTRITION

- Calories: 300
- Macros: 6g fat, 58g carbs, 7g protein

This hearty dish is warm and filling, creating a nutrient-packed breakfast rich in antioxidants, fiber, and anti-inflammatory compounds, supporting overall health and providing sustained energy.

Avocado Toast with Hemp Seeds, Arugula, and Poached Egg

DIRECTIONS

1. Toast bread, top with avocado, and add arugula.
2. Fill saucepan with 3-4 inches of water, add vinegar, and bring to a gentle boil.
3. Crack the egg into a small bowl.
4. Stir water to create a light whirlpool.
5. Gently slide egg into the water and cook 3-4 minutes until whites are set.
6. Lift the egg with a slotted spoon, drain excess water, and serve over toast.

INGREDIENTS

- 1 slice whole-grain bread
- ½ avocado, mashed
- 1 tbsp hemp seeds
- 1 cup arugula
- 1 fresh egg
- 1-2 tsp white vinegar (optional)
- Water

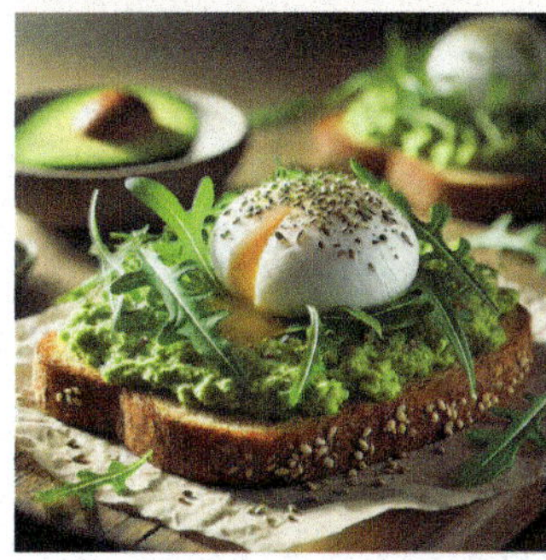

NUTRITION

- Calories: 300
- Macros: 18g fat, 30g carbs, 12g protein

Poaching an egg may take some practice, but the results are worth it for this tasty dish!

Quinoa Porridge with Almond Milk, Pecans, & Cooked Peaches

DIRECTIONS

1. Warm quinoa in almond milk until heated through.
2. In a separate pan, cook peaches with a splash of water and cinnamon until soft.
3. Top with cooked peaches, pecans, and cinnamon.

INGREDIENTS

- 1 cup cooked quinoa
- 1 cup almond milk
- 1 peach, diced
- ¼ cup pecans, chopped
- 1 tsp cinnamon

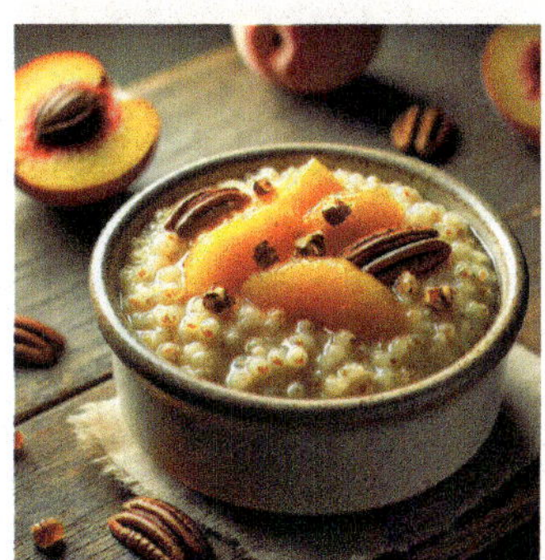

NUTRITION

- Calories: 350
- Macros: 15g fat, 48g carbs, 10g protein

Preparing the quinoa and cooking the peaches ahead of time for reheating shortens prep time for this delicious meal on a busy morning.

Sweet Potato and Spinach Hash with Poached Egg

INGREDIENTS

- 1 medium sweet potato, diced
- 1 cup spinach
- 1 egg
- 1 tbsp olive oil
- ½ tsp turmeric
- ½ tsp paprika
- Salt and pepper to taste

DIRECTIONS

1. Heat olive oil in a skillet and add diced sweet potatoes. Cook until tender.
2. Add spinach, turmeric, paprika, salt, and pepper, and sauté until spinach is wilted.
3. Poach the egg separately and serve on top of the hash.

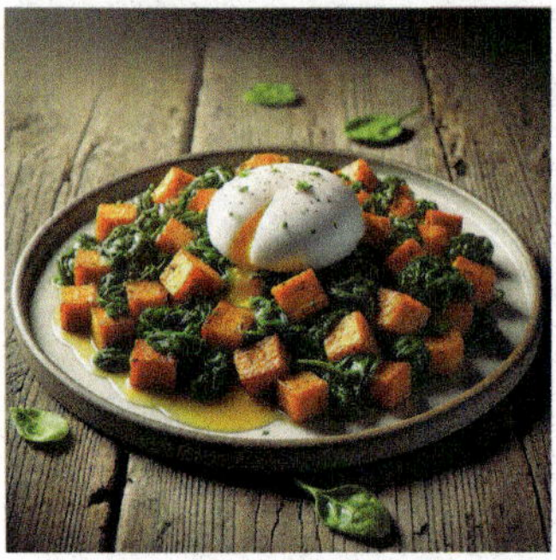

NUTRITION

- Calories: 280
- Macros: 14g fat, 32g carbs, 14g protein

This warm and filling breakfast incorporates turmeric for its flavor and anti-inflammatory properties.

Coconut Yogurt with Papaya, Chia Seeds, and Pistachios

INGREDIENTS

- 1 cup coconut yogurt
- ½ cup papaya, diced
- 1 tbsp chia seeds
- 2 tbsp pistachios, chopped

DIRECTIONS

1. Top coconut yogurt with diced papaya, chia seeds, and chopped pistachios.
2. Enjoy!

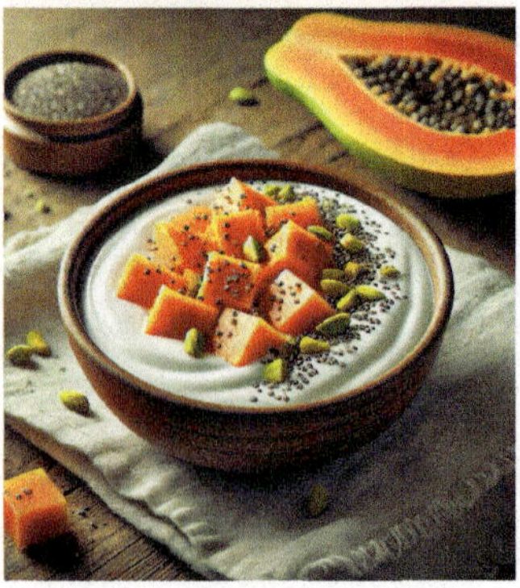

NUTRITION

- Calories: 250
- Macros: 14g fat, 28g carbs, 5g protein

Coconut yogurt is a dairy-free alternative to traditional yogurt, made from coconut milk instead of cow's milk. It's a popular choice for those who are lactose intolerant, vegan, or looking for a plant-based option.

Savory Oatmeal with Mushrooms, Spinach, and Walnuts

DIRECTIONS

1. Cook oats in water or broth until the mixture is creamy and the liquid is absorbed (about 5 minutes).
2. In a pan, sauté mushrooms in olive oil until tender.
3. Add spinach and sauté until wilted.
4. Stir into the oatmeal and top with chopped walnuts.

INGREDIENTS

- ½ cup rolled oats
- 1 cup water or vegetable broth
- ½ cup mushrooms, sliced
- 1 cup spinach
- 1 tbsp olive oil
- 2 tbsp walnuts, chopped
- Salt and pepper

NUTRITION

- Calories: 280
- Macros: 14g fat, 35g carbs, 8g protein

This savory take on oatmeal offers another delicious way to enjoy this hearty meal option.

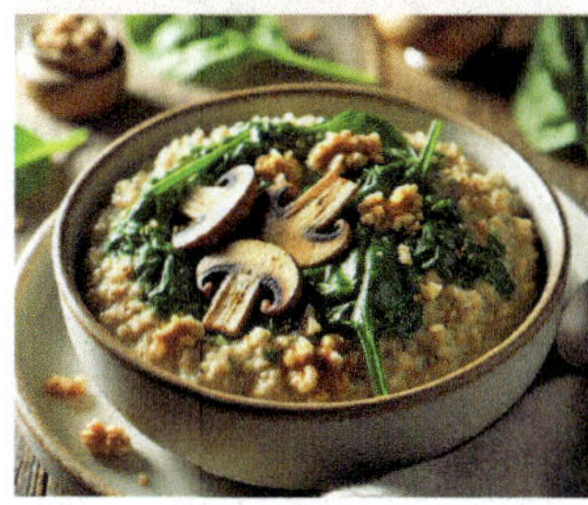

Blueberry and Flaxseed Smoothie with Ginger

DIRECTIONS

1. Place blueberries, flaxseeds, ginger, almond milk, and banana into a blender.
2. Blend until smooth.
3. Serve immediately and enjoy!

INGREDIENTS

- 1 cup frozen blueberries
- 1 tbsp flaxseeds
- 1 tsp fresh ginger, grated
- 1 cup unsweetened almond milk
- 1 banana

NUTRITION

- Calories: 250
- Macros: 6g fat, 45g carbs, 5g protein

Smoothies are a quick and convenient way to get essential nutrients, especially on busy mornings when time is limited.

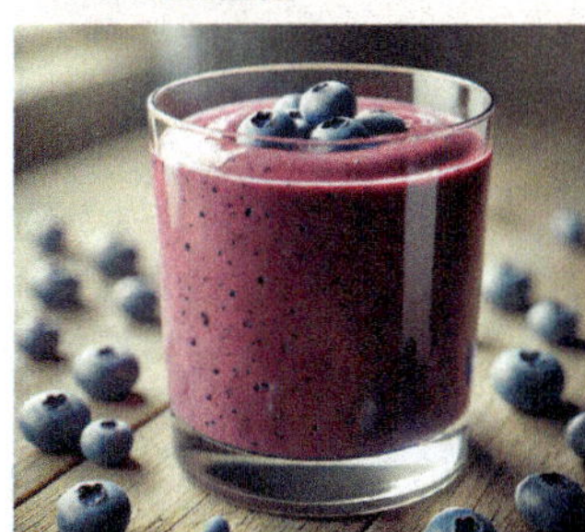

Millet Porridge with Coconut Milk, Berries, and Almonds

INGREDIENTS

- ½ cup millet, rinsed
- 1 cup coconut milk
- ½ cup mixed berries
- 2 tbsp almonds, chopped
- 1 tsp honey (optional)

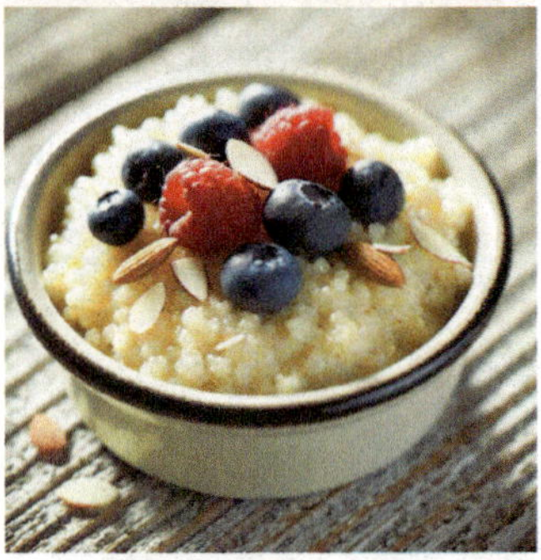

DIRECTIONS

1. Place millet and coconut milk in a saucepan over medium heat.
2. Cook, stirring frequently, until soft and creamy.
3. Top with berries, almonds, and a drizzle of honey.

NUTRITION

- Calories: 300
- Macros: 14g fat, 45g carbs, 6g protein

Millet is a versatile, gluten-free ancient grain, rich in nutrients, including fiber, protein, and essential minerals, making it a healthy and sustainable alternative to other grains like rice or wheat.

Amaranth Porridge with Pear, Cinnamon, and Walnuts

INGREDIENTS

- ½ cup amaranth
- 1 cup water or almond milk
- 1 pear, sliced
- 1 tsp cinnamon
- 2 tbsp walnuts, chopped
- Drizzle of honey or maple syrup

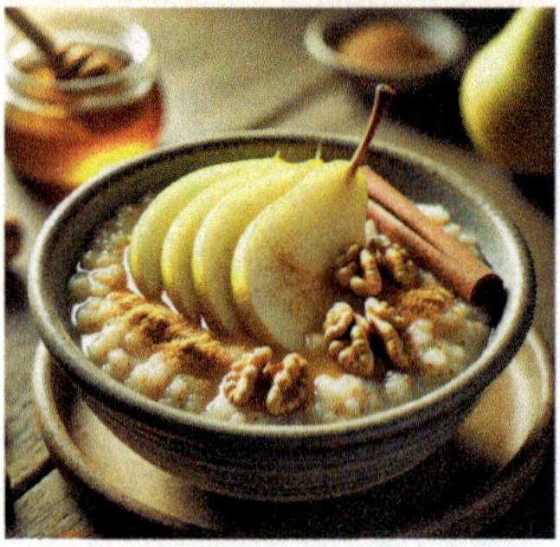

DIRECTIONS

1. Cook amaranth in water or almond milk until tender and liquid is absorbed.
2. Top with sliced pear, cinnamon, and walnuts.
3. Drizzle with honey or maple syrup if desired.

NUTRITION

- Calories: 280
- Macros: 10g fat, 50g carbs, 8g protein

Amaranth is a nutrient-dense, gluten-free grain, high in protein, fiber, and essential amino acids, making it ideal for a balanced and healthy diet.

Overnight Oats with Chia Seeds, Blueberries, and Maple Syrup

DIRECTIONS

1. In a jar, combine oats, chia seeds, almond milk, and cinnamon. Stir well.
2. Cover and refrigerate overnight.
3. In the morning, top with blueberries and drizzle with maple syrup.
4. You can enjoy our overnight oats cold, straight from the fridge, or warm them up slightly if preferred.

INGREDIENTS

- ½ cup rolled oats
- 1 tbsp chia seeds
- 1 cup unsweetened almond milk (or milk of choice)
- ¼ tsp cinnamon
- ½ cup fresh blueberries
- 1 tsp maple syrup

NUTRITION

- Calories: 280
- Macros: 9g fat, 43g carbs, 7g protein

This recipe is perfect for busy mornings, providing a delicious, nutritious, and easy start to your day. You can swap out different toppings for variety.

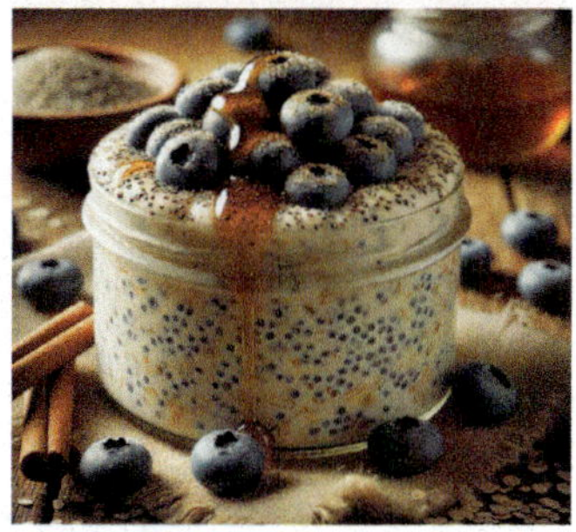

Green Smoothie with Berries and Banana

DIRECTIONS

1. Add all ingredients to a blender.
2. Blend until smooth.
3. Serve immediately.
4. Enjoy!

INGREDIENTS

- 1 cup spinach
- 1 cup frozen mixed berries
- 1 banana
- 1 tbsp flaxseeds
- 1 cup unsweetened almond milk

NUTRITION

- Calories: 250
- Macros: 6g fat, 48g carbs, 5g protein

This green smoothie is a quick, nutritious way to start your day or boost your energy anytime!

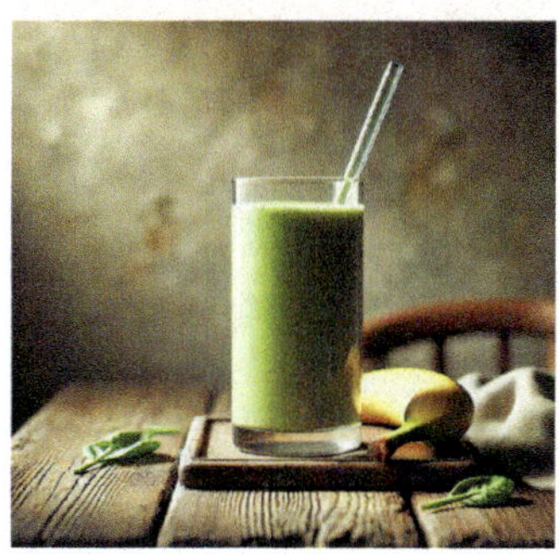

Acai Bowl with Banana, Granola, Chia Seeds, & Fresh Berries

INGREDIENTS

- 1 frozen acai berry smoothie packet
- 1 banana
- ½ cup almond milk
- ½ cup mixed berries
- ¼ cup granola
- 1 tbsp chia seeds

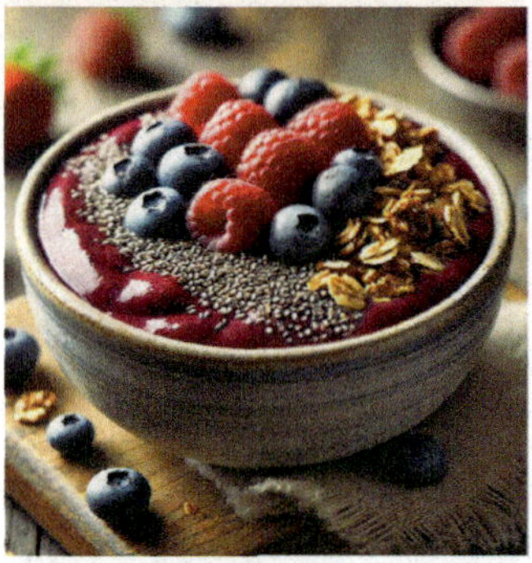

DIRECTIONS

1. Blend the acai packet, banana, and almond milk until smooth.
2. Pour into a bowl and top with granola, chia seeds, and fresh berries.

NUTRITION

- Calories: 350
- Macros: 12g fat, 60g carbs, 6g protein

This is a quick and easy choice for a nutritious start to your day. You can use whichever milk you choose and vary your toppings.

Turmeric & Cinnamon Millet Porridge with Apples and Pecans

INGREDIENTS

- ½ cup millet
- 1 cup almond milk
- 1 apple, diced
- 1 tsp cinnamon
- ½ tsp turmeric
- 2 tbsp pecans

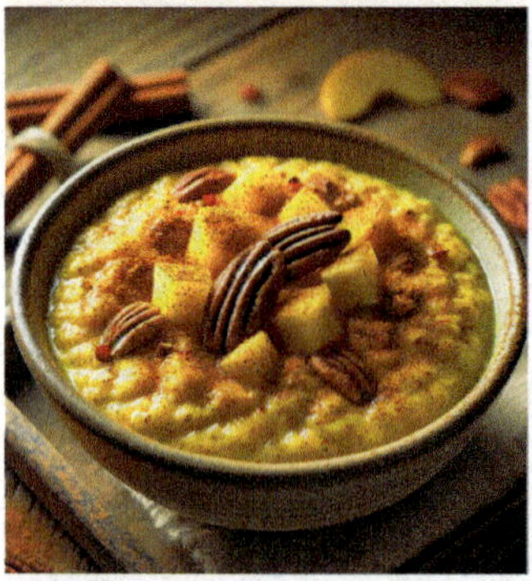

DIRECTIONS

1. Cook millet in almond milk until tender and liquid is absorbed.
2. Transfer to a bowl.
3. Top with diced apple, cinnamon, turmeric, and halved or chopped pecans.

NUTRITION

- Calories: 320
- Macros: 14g fat, 45g carbs, 8g protein

The delicious combination of the anti-inflammatory spices turmeric and cinnamon helps to reduce inflammation and support immune health, making this a soothing and nutritious meal.

Buckwheat Pancakes with Blueberries and Maple Syrup

DIRECTIONS

1. Mix buckwheat flour, egg, almond milk, and baking powder to form a batter.
2. Cook pancakes on a non-stick skillet until golden.
3. Top with blueberries and maple syrup.

INGREDIENTS

- ½ cup buckwheat flour
- 1 egg
- ½ cup almond milk
- 1 tsp baking powder
- ½ cup fresh blueberries
- 2 tbsp maple syrup

NUTRITION

- Calories: 300
- Macros: 10g fat, 45g carbs, 10g protein

This nutritious, gluten-free breakfast is packed with fiber, antioxidants, and anti-inflammatory properties, making it a wholesome and delicious breakfast.

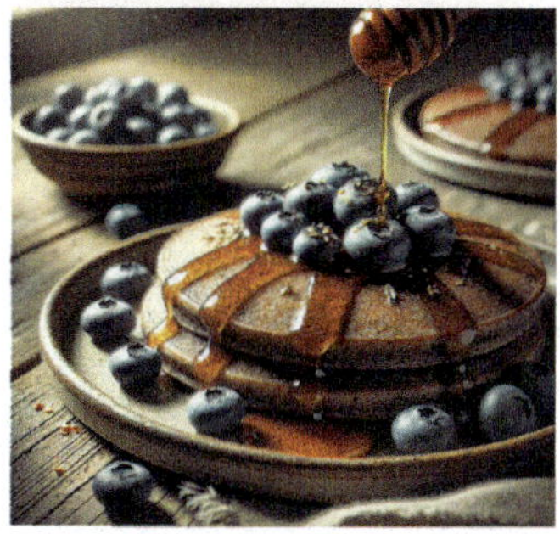

Oatmeal with Pear, Almonds, and a Drizzle of Honey

DIRECTIONS

1. Cook oats in almond milk until tender and liquid is absorbed.
2. Transfer to a bowl.
3. Top with diced pear, almonds, and a drizzle of honey.
4. Serve hot and enjoy!

INGREDIENTS

- ½ cup rolled oats
- 1 cup almond milk
- 1 pear, diced
- 2 tbsp almonds, whole, slivered, or chopped
- 1 tsp honey

NUTRITION

- Calories: 320
- Macros: 12g fat, 50g carbs, 8g protein

This delicious, hearty breakfast is rich in fiber, healthy fats, and natural antioxidants, providing a balanced start to your day with anti-inflammatory benefits.

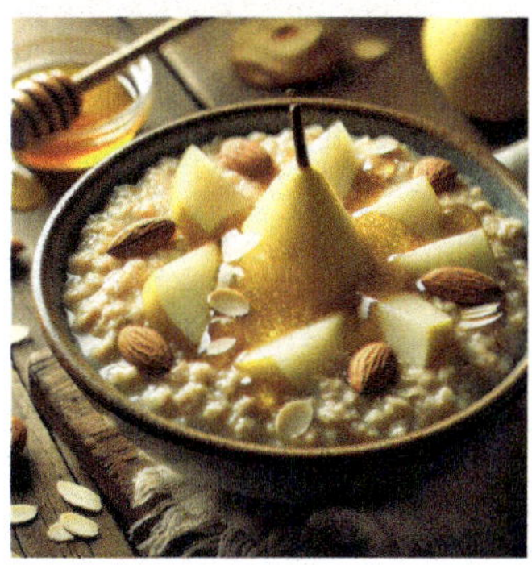

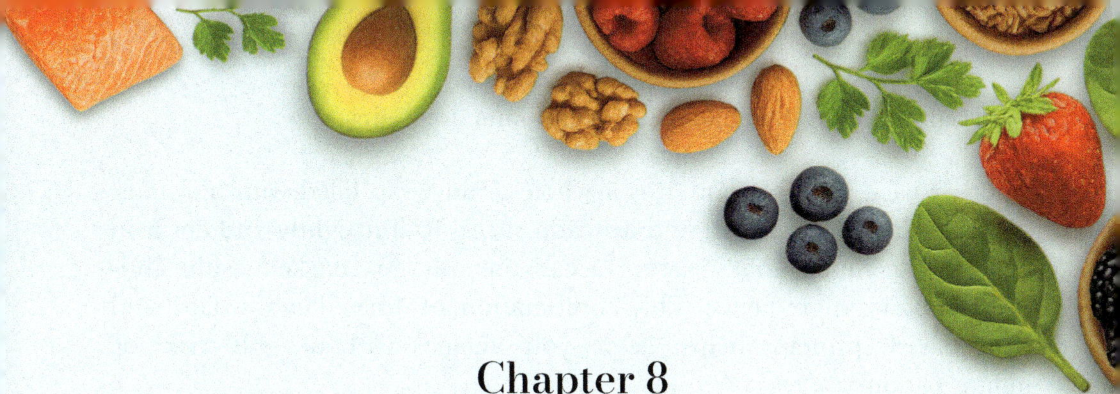

Chapter 8

Satisfying Anti-Inflammatory Lunches

In the tapestry of daily eating, lunch occupies a pivotal space, a midday pause that can either restore energy and focus or leave us feeling sluggish and inflamed. This meal, often squeezed between meetings or errands, holds the quiet power to sway the day's rhythm, tipping the scales toward sustained vitality or toward the lull of afternoon fatigue.

Busy mornings often leave little time for elaborate meal prep. However, nourishing meals that support our health goals are still essential. Whether juggling a demanding office job or moving through a busy class schedule, having simple, prepared lunches can be a game-changer. The secret is in simplicity and a little preparation.

Consider assembling a colorful salad with mixed greens, cherry tomatoes, sliced cucumbers, and a handful of walnuts, all topped with a light lemon-olive oil dressing. Prepare this the night before, store it in an airtight container, keep the dressing separate, and it's ready to grab on your way out the door. For added protein, toss in some wild-caught salmon or slices of grilled chicken if you wish.

Another easy, portable option is a whole-grain wrap filled with hummus, spinach, shredded carrots, and avocado slices. Roll it tightly and cut it in half for a lunch that's easy to eat on the go, packed with anti-inflammatory ingredients. This combination of fiber, healthy fats, and plant-based protein helps keep you fueled without the risk of inflammation.

Quick Home Lunches

For those with access to a kitchen at lunchtime, the possibilities expand. A quick sauté of quinoa, black beans, bell peppers, and onions, seasoned with cumin and coriander, makes for a fast, nutritious meal. Topped with a dollop of Greek yogurt and a squeeze of lime, this dish provides ample protein and fiber. It offers added anti-inflammatory benefits from the spices.

Another quick option is a roasted tomato, garlic, and red pepper soup, blended until smooth and served with a slice of toasted whole-grain bread. This comforting soup delivers antioxidants from tomatoes, allicin from garlic, and capsaicin from red peppers, all known for their anti-inflammatory effects, while the whole-grain bread adds a satisfying crunch.

Utilizing Leftovers

Leftovers make excellent lunches that are both quick and versatile. Roasted chicken, sweet potatoes, and broccoli from dinner can easily transform into a vibrant lunch bowl. Shred the chicken, chop the vegetables, and layer them over mixed greens. Add avocado slices and a sprinkle of seeds—pumpkin, sunflower, or chia—for added texture and healthy fats. A simple vinaigrette made with olive oil, balsamic vinegar, mustard, and honey ties everything together with a boost of flavor and health benefits.

For a creative spin, turn leftover grilled vegetables into a frittata. Beat a few eggs, pour over the veggies in a hot skillet, and let it set. Adding a touch of turmeric enhances the dish's anti-inflammatory properties. This meal, paired with a side of mixed berries, combines protein, fiber, antioxidants, and healthy fats for a lunch that keeps you energized all afternoon.

Thermos-Friendly Soups and Stews

Soups and stews offer warmth and comfort while delivering essential nutrients. A thermos of lentil soup simmered with tomatoes, onions, and spices like cumin, coriander, and cinnamon provides a nourishing meal rich in protein and antioxidants. Perfect for hectic days, it keeps its heat and offers a soothing, health-boosting lunch.

A hearty chicken and vegetable stew, thickened with sweet potatoes and flavored with rosemary and thyme, provides a meal full of complex carbohydrates and anti-inflammatory herbs. It's a perfect example of how slow cooking deepens flavors, creating a satisfying lunch to enjoy whenever your schedule allows.

Snack Boxes

For those days when traditional meals aren't possible, snack boxes provide a practical alternative. Fill them with almonds, carrot sticks, pear slices, hummus with cucumber rounds, or a few squares of dark chocolate with walnuts. These quick, nutrient-dense snacks are easy to eat on the go, helping you stay on track with your anti-inflammatory diet, even during the busiest moments.

Basic Grains

The first two recipes in this section are for basic quinoa and brown rice. They are excellent staples in an anti-inflammatory diet, providing fiber, essential minerals, and plant-based protein that support digestion, blood sugar stability, and overall health. These versatile, fiber-rich grains work well as the foundation for a variety of meals, from hearty grain bowls to side dishes for protein-rich entrees.

Preparing batches of quinoa and brown rice at the start of each week saves time and ensures you have a nutritious base ready to go. This meal prep approach makes it easy to create balanced lunches and dinners by simply adding fresh or roasted vegetables, lean proteins, and healthy fats. Quinoa's slightly nutty flavor and brown rice's satisfying chew add variety and texture, helping to keep meals interesting and nourishing throughout the week.

Anti-Inflammatory Lunch Recipes

The following recipes offer a range of flavors and complexity, catering to various tastes, dietary needs, and culinary skills. Feel free to explore these options and create meal plans tailored to your preferences. Whether prepared in the calm of the morning, during a break in your busy workday, or with fresh leftovers, these healthy lunches provide a nourishing midday break that supports your well-being, boosts your energy, and satisfies your palate.

Basic Fluffy Quinoa

DIRECTIONS

1. Place the quinoa in a fine-mesh strainer and rinse under cold water to remove the natural coating (saponin), which can make quinoa taste bitter.
2. Bring the water or broth, oil, and salt to a boil in a medium saucepan.
3. Add quinoa, cover, and simmer for about 15 minutes, or until liquid is absorbed.
4. Remove saucepan from heat and let it stand, covered for 5 minutes, then fluff with a fork.
5. You can double or triple the recipe for meal prep if desired.

NUTRITION

- Calories (per 1 cup serving): 222
- Macros: 4g fat, 39g carbs, 8g protein

INGREDIENTS

- 1 cup quinoa
- 2 cups water or vegetable broth (for extra flavor)
- 1 tsp olive oil
- ¼ tsp salt

This recipe yields about 3 cups of light and fluffy quinoa. It can be made ahead and rewarmed to make your meal prep or weeknight dinners easier.

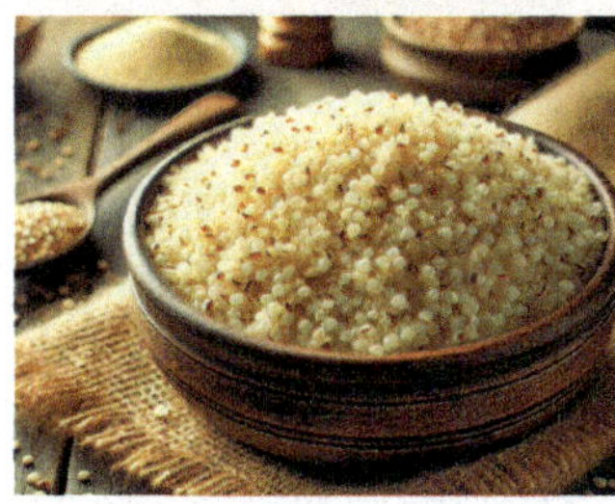

Basic Brown Rice

DIRECTIONS

1. Rinse rice under cold water in a fine-mesh strainer to remove excess starch.
2. Bring water or broth and salt to a boil in a medium saucepan.
3. Add rice, stir once, reduce heat to low, cover, and simmer 40-45 minutes, or until liquid is absorbed and rice is tender.
4. Remove from heat, let stand, covered, for 5-10 minutes, then fluff with a fork.
5. You can double or triple the recipe for meal prep if desired.

NUTRITION

- Calories (per 1 cup serving): 220
- Macros: 2g fat, 45g carbs, 5g protein

INGREDIENTS

- 1 cup brown rice
- 2 cups water (or vegetable broth for added flavor)
- ½ tsp salt

This easy recipe makes about 3 cups of rice and is great for meal prep. It can be made ahead to provide a nutritious base for many meals.

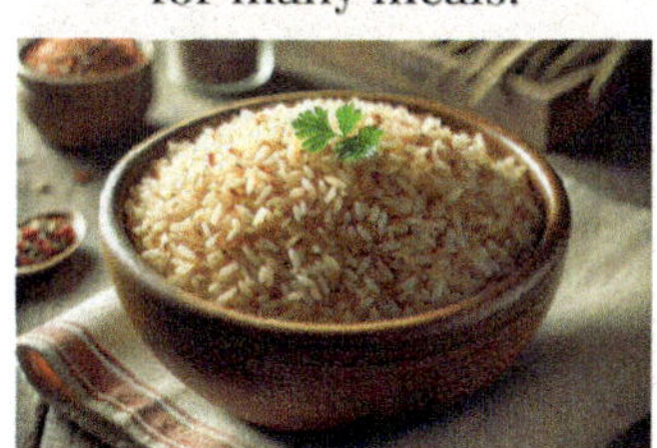

Quinoa and Chickpea Salad with Lemon-Tahini Dressing

INGREDIENTS

- 1 cup cooked quinoa
- ½ cup canned chickpeas, rinsed and drained
- ½ cucumber, diced
- ½ cup sliced tomatoes
- ¼ red onion, thinly sliced
- 2 tbsp fresh parsley, chopped

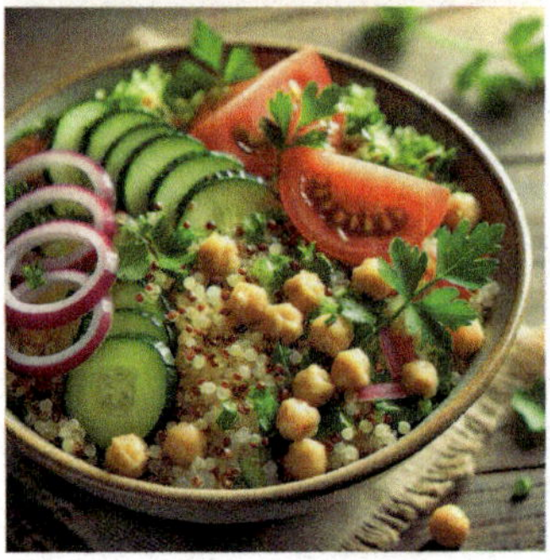

LEMON-TAHINI DRESSING

- 1 tbsp tahini
- 1 tbsp olive oil
- 1 tbsp lemon juice
- 1 tsp honey
- 1 clove garlic, minced
- Salt and pepper to taste

DIRECTIONS

1. In a large bowl, combine quinoa, chickpeas, cucumber, tomatoes, red onion, and parsley.
2. In a small bowl, whisk together the dressing ingredients.
3. Pour dressing over the salad and toss to combine.

NUTRITION

- Calories: 400
- Macros: 17g fat, 55g carbs, 13g protein

This refreshing salad is easy to prepare, and is a filling and enjoyable lunch.

Lentil and Vegetable Soup

INGREDIENTS

- 1 cup lentils, rinsed
- 1 carrot, diced
- 2 celery stalks, diced
- 1 onion, diced
- 3 cups vegetable broth
- 1 tsp turmeric
- 1 tsp cumin
- Salt and pepper

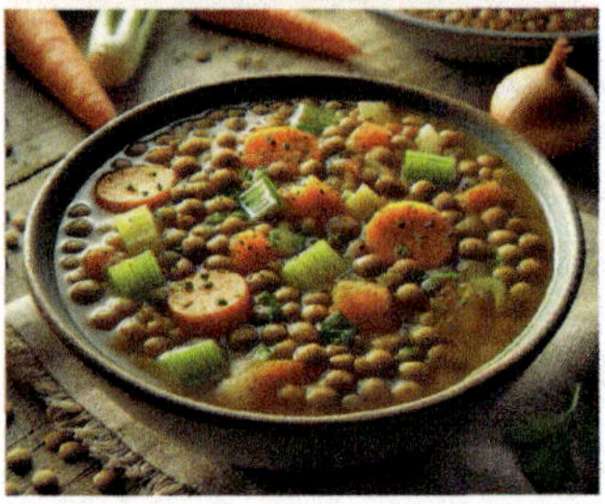

DIRECTIONS

1. In a large pot, sauté the onion, carrot, and celery in olive oil until softened.
2. Add lentils, vegetable broth, turmeric, cumin, salt, and pepper.
3. Simmer for 25-30 minutes until lentils are tender.
4. Serve hot, and enjoy!

NUTRITION

- Calories: 350
- Macros: 3g fat, 55g carbs, 20g protein

This hearty soup can be made ahead and the left-overs can be frozen or prepped for additional lunches or a quick dinner.

Sweet Potato and Black Bean Tacos

DIRECTIONS

1. Preheat oven to 400°F (200°C).
2. Toss peeled and diced sweet potatoes with olive oil and spices.
3. Spread on a lined baking sheet and roast for 25-30 minutes, until tender.
4. Drain and rinse black beans, then heat in a small saucepan.
5. Warm tortillas in a dry skillet.
6. Add sweet potatoes, black beans, avocado, and cilantro to each tortilla.
7. Serve immediately.

INGREDIENTS

- 2 medium sweet potatoes
- 1 can (15 oz) black beans
- 1 tsp cumin
- 1 tsp chili powder
- 2 tbsp olive oil
- 8 small corn tortillas
- ½ avocado, sliced
- ¼ cup fresh cilantro, chopped
- Salt and pepper

NUTRITION

- Calories: 450
- Macros: 16g fat, 68g carbs, 12g protein

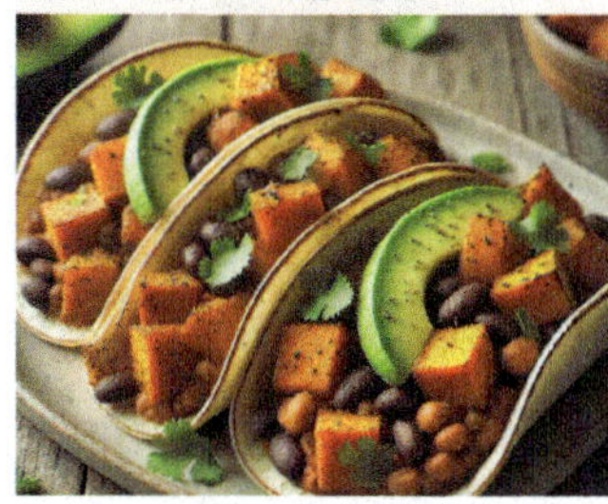

These vegan tacos offer a delicious combination of fiber, plant-based protein, and anti-inflammatory spices.

Tuna Salad with Olive Oil and Fresh Herbs

DIRECTIONS

1. In a bowl, mix the drained tuna with olive oil, lemon juice, parsley, dill, salt, and pepper.
2. Serve the tuna salad over a bed of mixed greens.
3. Enjoy immediately or refrigerate for later.

INGREDIENTS

- 1 can (5 oz) tuna in water, drained
- 2 tbsp olive oil
- 1 tbsp lemon juice
- 1 tbsp fresh parsley, chopped
- 1 tbsp fresh dill, chopped
- 1 cup mixed greens
- Salt and pepper

NUTRITION

- Calories: 320
- Macros: 22g fat, 2g carbs, 28g protein

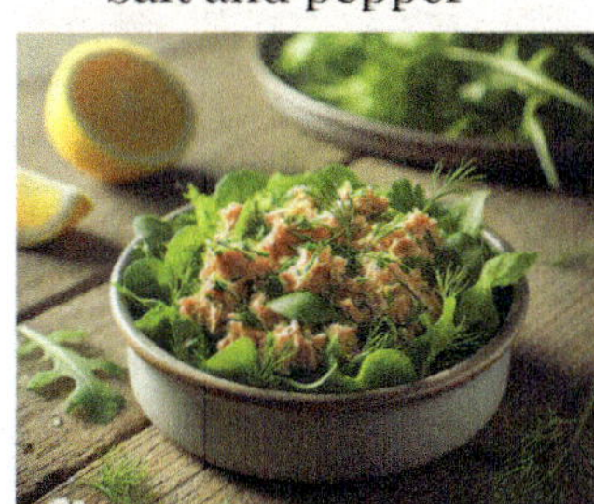

A refreshing, protein-rich salad made with heart-healthy olive oil and herbs, perfect for an anti-inflammatory lunch.

Avocado and Hummus Veggie Wrap

INGREDIENTS

- 1 whole-grain wrap or tortilla
- ¼ cup hummus
- ½ avocado, sliced
- ½ cup spinach
- ¼ cup shredded carrots
- ¼ cup cucumber slices
- Salt and pepper

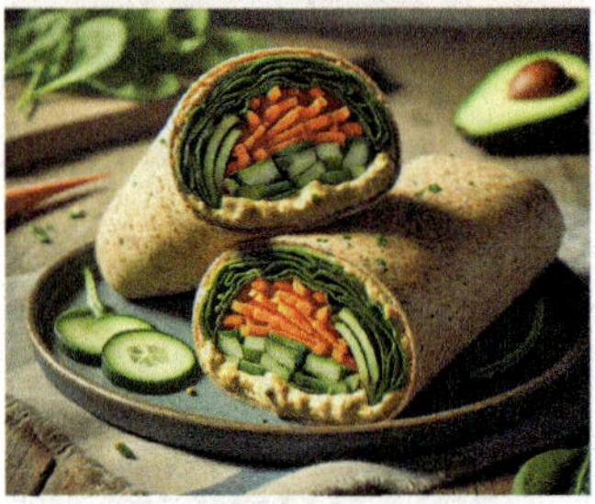

DIRECTIONS

1. Spread the hummus evenly over the whole-grain wrap.
2. Layer the avocado slices, spinach, carrots, and cucumber on top.
3. Sprinkle with salt and pepper to taste.
4. Roll the wrap tightly, cut in half, and serve immediately.

NUTRITION

- Calories: 380
- Macros: 22g fat, 40g carbs, 8g protein

This easy-to-assemble wrap is packed with fiber, healthy fats, and antioxidants, making it a quick, anti-inflammatory meal.

Roasted Chickpea, Quinoa, and Veggie Bowl

INGREDIENTS

- 1 can (15 oz) chickpeas
- 1 cup cooked quinoa
- 1 cup spinach
- ½ cup cubed sweet potatoes
- ½ avocado, sliced
- 3 tbsp olive oil
- 1-2 tbsp Lemon Tahini dressing (see chapter 6)
- Salt and pepper

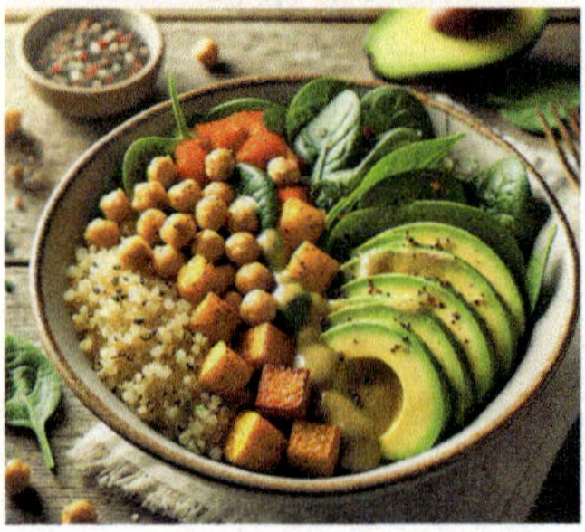

DIRECTIONS

1. Preheat oven to 400°F (200°C).
2. Drain and rinse chickpeas, then toss with sweet potatoes in 2 tbsp olive oil, cumin, salt, and pepper.
3. Roast on a lined sheet pan for 25-30 minutes until chickpeas are crispy and sweet potatoes are soft.
4. Arrange quinoa, spinach, roasted sweet potatoes, and avocado in a bowl.
5. Top with roasted chickpeas and Lemon Tahini dressing before serving.

NUTRITION

- Calories: 520
- Macros: 24g fat, 60g carbs, 15g protein

This nutrient-dense bowl combines roasted chickpeas, fresh veggies, and quinoa for a hearty, anti-inflammatory meal.

Chicken and Avocado Salad

INGREDIENTS

- 2 cooked chicken breasts, shredded
- 1 avocado, sliced
- 1 cup mixed greens
- ½ cup cherry tomatoes, halved
- 2 tbsp olive oil
- Juice of 1 lime
- Salt and pepper

DIRECTIONS

1. In a large bowl, combine the shredded chicken, sliced avocado, mixed greens, and cherry tomatoes.
2. In a small bowl, whisk together olive oil, lime juice, salt, and pepper.
3. Drizzle the dressing over the salad and toss to coat.
4. Serve immediately.

NUTRITION

- Calories: 430
- Macros: 28g fat, 12g carbs, 33g protein

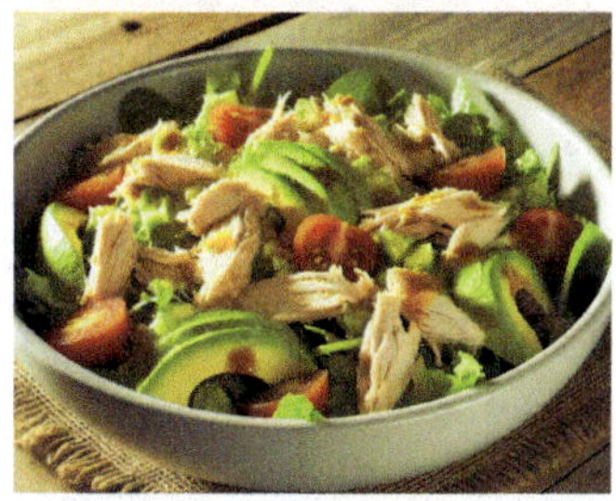

This protein-packed salad combines tender chicken with creamy avocado, providing protein, healthy fats, and anti-inflammatory benefits.

Eggplant and Zucchini Gratin

INGREDIENTS

- 1 medium eggplant
- 2 medium zucchinis
- 1 cup marinara sauce (see chapter 6)
- 2 tbsp olive oil
- 2 cloves garlic, minced
- ¼ cup grated Parmesan cheese (optional)
- Salt and pepper

DIRECTIONS

1. Preheat oven to 375°F (190°C). Grease a baking dish with olive oil.
2. In a skillet, sauté garlic in olive oil for 1-2 minutes.
3. Layer eggplant and zucchini slices in the dish, alternating between them.
4. Pour marinara sauce over the vegetables and sprinkle with Parmesan cheese if using.
5. Bake for 25-30 minutes until the vegetables are tender.

NUTRITION

- Calories: 290
- Macros: 17g fat, 30g carbs, 7g protein

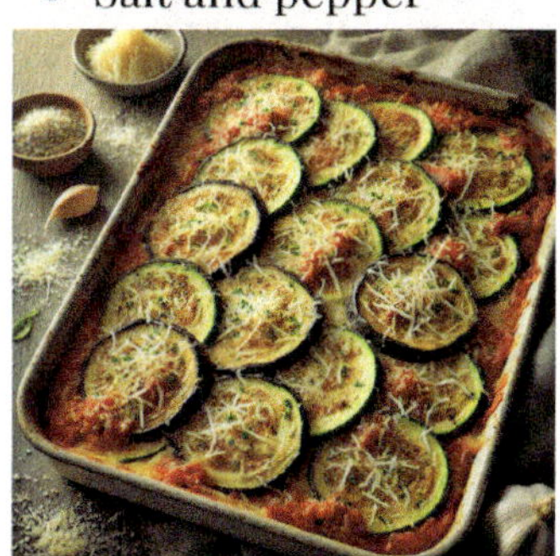

This baked gratin combines the anti-inflammatory power of olive oil and garlic with nutritious eggplant and zucchini.

Rainbow Veggie Buddha Bowl

INGREDIENTS

- ½ cup cooked brown rice
- ¼ cup chickpeas
- ¼ cup shredded carrots
- ¼ cup red cabbage, shredded
- ¼ cup cucumber, sliced
- ¼ cup cherry tomatoes, halved
- 2 tbsp Lemon Tahini dressing (see chapter 6)

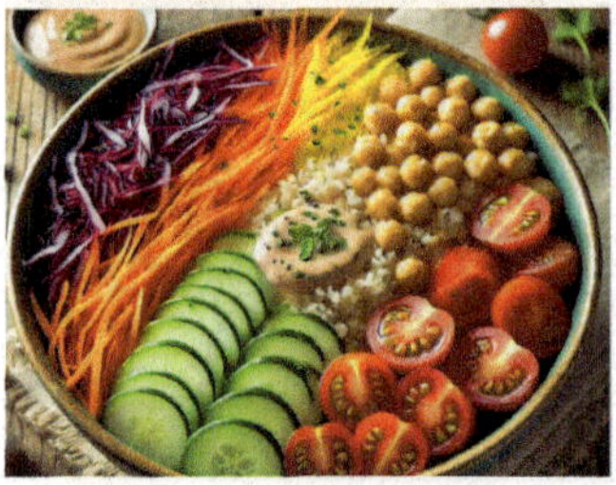

DIRECTIONS

1. Cook brown rice according to package directions (May be prepped ahead of time).
2. Arrange brown rice, chickpeas (drained and rinsed), carrots, cabbage, cucumber, and cherry tomatoes in a bowl.
3. Top the bowl with Lemon Tahini dressing and enjoy.

NUTRITION

- Calories: 350
- Macros: 22g fat, 15g carbs, 25g protein

This colorful bowl is a balanced, anti-inflammatory lunch, rich in fiber and antioxidants.

Spinach and Quinoa Salad with Pomegranate and Pecans

INGREDIENTS

- 2 cups spinach
- ½ cup cooked quinoa
- ¼ cup pomegranate seeds
- 2 tbsp pecans (halved or chopped)
- 1 tbsp balsamic vinaigrette

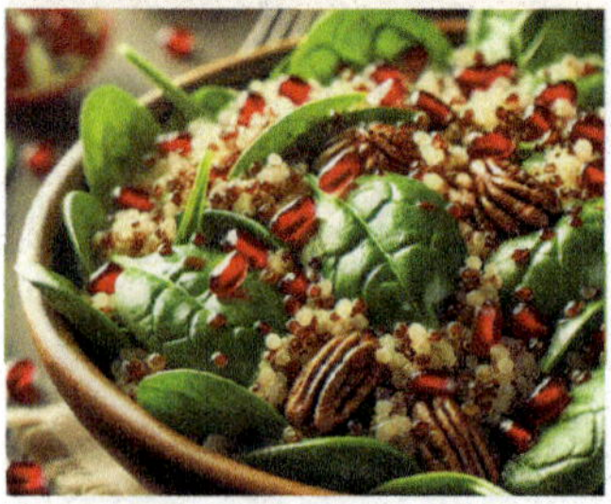

DIRECTIONS

1. Toss spinach, pomegranate seeds, and cooked quinoa in a bowl with balsamic vinaigrette.
2. Top with pecans for added protein and crunch.
3. Enjoy!

NUTRITION

- Calories: 300
- Macros: 8g fat, 30g carbs, 18g protein

This vibrant salad is packed with antioxidants, fiber, and healthy fats, offering a delicious blend of flavors and anti-inflammatory benefits.

Hummus, Veggie, and Quinoa Wrap

DIRECTIONS

1. Spread hummus evenly over the whole-grain wrap.
2. Add quinoa, shredded carrots, cucumber slices, and spinach.
3. Sprinkle with salt and pepper.
4. Roll the wrap tightly, cut in half, and enjoy.

INGREDIENTS

- 1 whole-grain wrap or tortilla
- ¼ cup cooked quinoa
- ¼ cup hummus
- ½ cup shredded carrots
- ½ cup cucumber slices
- ¼ cup spinach
- Salt and pepper

NUTRITION

- Calories: 370
- Macros: 14g fat, 50g carbs, 12g protein

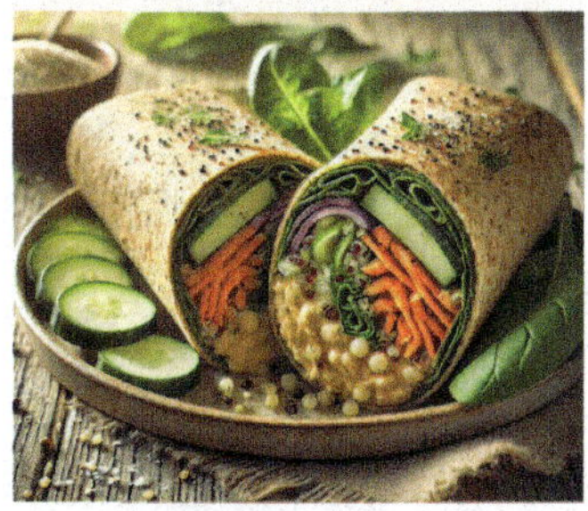

The fiber-rich quinoa, crunchy veggies, and creamy hummus, makes this wrap satisfying, anti-inflammatory, and packed with plant-based protein.

Spinach and Lentil Salad with Pomegranate Seeds

DIRECTIONS

1. In a large bowl, combine cooked lentils, spinach, pomegranate seeds, and walnuts.
2. Add balsamic vinaigrette dressing just before serving, and toss well to coat.
3. Enjoy.

INGREDIENTS

- 1 cup cooked lentils
- 2 cups fresh spinach
- ¼ cup pomegranate seeds
- ¼ cup chopped walnuts
- 2-3 tbsp balsamic vinaigrette (see chapter 6)
- Salt and pepper

NUTRITION

- Calories: 400
- Macros: 23g fat, 40g carbs, 15g protein

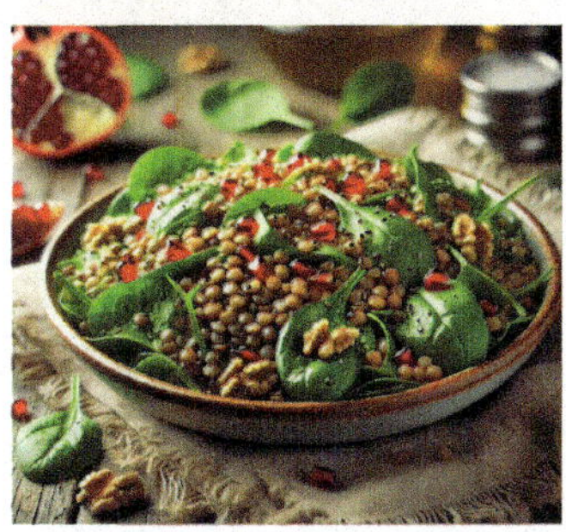

This hearty salad is rich in fiber, protein, and antioxidants from lentils and pomegranate seeds, making it a powerful anti-inflammatory meal.

Curried Chickpea and Sweet Potato Stew

INGREDIENTS

- 1 can (15 oz) chickpeas
- 1 medium sweet potato, peeled and diced
- 1 cup coconut milk
- 1 cup vegetable broth
- 1 tbsp curry powder
- 1 tsp turmeric
- 2 cloves garlic, minced
- 2 tbsp olive oil
- Salt and pepper

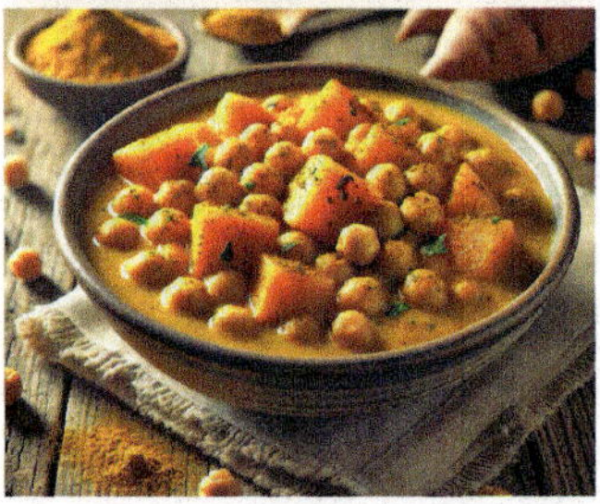

DIRECTIONS

1. Heat olive oil in a large pot.
2. Add garlic and cook for 1-2 minutes.
3. Stir in diced sweet potato, curry powder, turmeric, and chickpeas (drained and rinsed). Cook for 5 minutes.
4. Add coconut milk and vegetable broth. Bring to a simmer and cook for 15-20 minutes, until the sweet potatoes are tender.
5. Season with salt and pepper, and serve warm.

NUTRITION

- Calories: 450
- Macros: 22g fat, 52g carbs, 12g protein

This hearty, warming stew is rich in anti-inflammatory spices like turmeric and curry, paired with filling ingredients.

Quinoa Salad with Avocado, Spinach, and Cherry Tomatoes

INGREDIENTS

- 1 cup cooked quinoa
- 1 cup fresh spinach
- 1 avocado, sliced
- 1 cup cherry tomatoes, halved
- 2 tbsp olive oil
- Juice of 1 lemon
- Salt and pepper

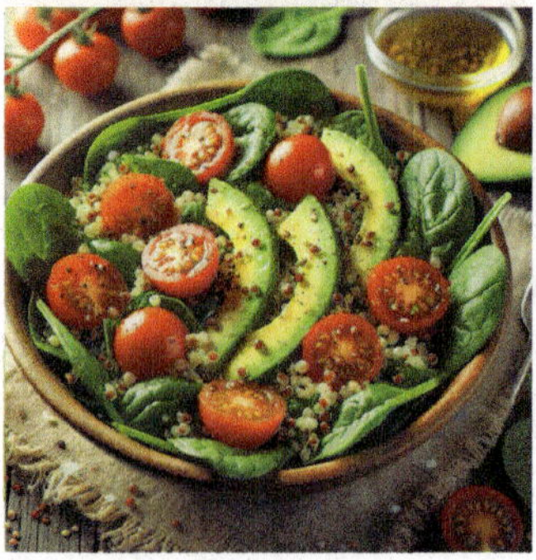

DIRECTIONS

1. In a large bowl, combine the cooked quinoa, fresh spinach, avocado, and cherry tomatoes.
2. In a small bowl, whisk together the olive oil, lemon juice, salt, and pepper.
3. Pour the dressing over the quinoa mixture and toss until everything is well coated.
4. Serve immediately or store in the fridge for up to 24 hours.

NUTRITION

- Calories: 420
- Macros: 25g fat, 45g carbs, 8g protein

A fresh and vibrant quinoa salad packed with fiber, healthy fats, and antioxidants to keep inflammation at bay.

Kale and Sweet Potato Soup

INGREDIENTS

- 2 medium sweet potatoes, peeled and diced
- 2 cups kale, chopped
- 1 onion, chopped
- 2 cloves garlic, minced
- 4 cups vegetable broth
- 1 tsp turmeric
- 1 tsp cumin
- 2 tbsp olive oil
- Salt and pepper

DIRECTIONS

1. Heat olive oil in a large pot over medium heat. Add onion and garlic, and sauté for 3-4 minutes.
2. Stir in sweet potatoes, turmeric, cumin, and vegetable broth. Bring to a boil, then reduce heat and simmer for 20 minutes.
3. Add kale and cook for another 5 minutes until the sweet potatoes are tender and kale is wilted.
4. Season with salt and pepper.
5. Serve hot.

NUTRITION

- Calories: 300
- Macros: 12g fat, 44g carbs, 5g protein

This hearty soup combines kale, sweet potatoes, and anti-inflammatory spices for a warming, nutrient-rich lunch.

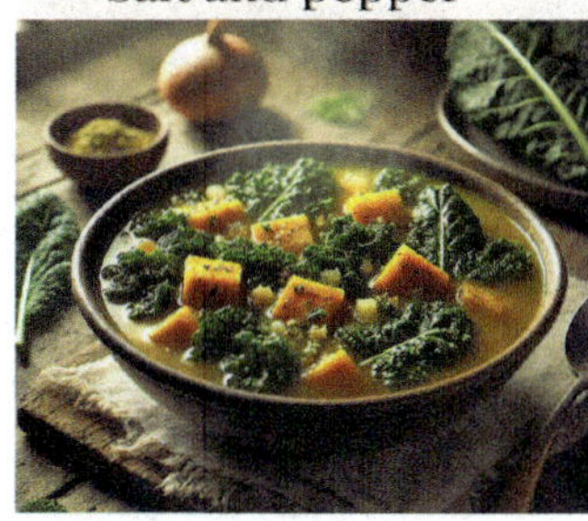

Spinach and Strawberry Salad

INGREDIENTS

- 2 cups spinach
- ½ cup strawberries, sliced
- ¼ cup walnuts, whole or chopped
- 1-2 tbsp balsamic vinaigrette (see chapter 6)

DIRECTIONS

1. Toss spinach, sliced strawberries, and walnuts together in a bowl.
2. Drizzle with balsamic vinaigrette before serving.
3. Enjoy!

NUTRITION

- Calories: 250
- Macros: 18g fat, 22g carbs, 6g protein

This salad is rich in fiber and healthy fats, offering a filling anti-inflammatory option for lunch.

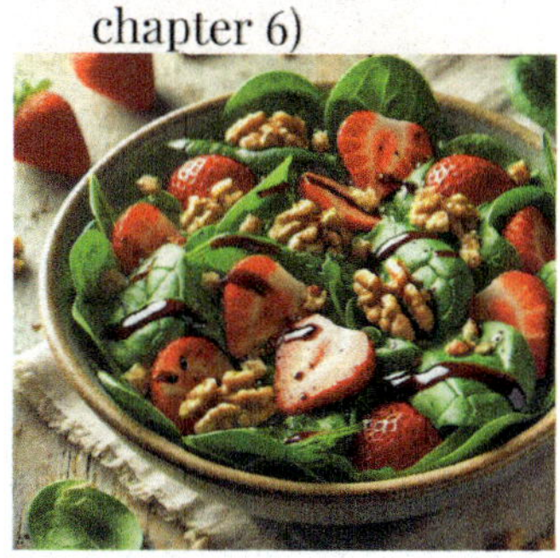

Lentil and Sweet Potato Salad

INGREDIENTS

- 1 medium sweet potato, diced
- 1 cup lentils, cooked according to package directions
- 1 cup spinach
- 2 tbsp olive oil
- 1 tsp cumin
- 1 tbsp lemon juice
- Salt and pepper to taste

DIRECTIONS

1. Preheat oven to 400°F (200°C).
2. Toss diced sweet potatoes with 1 tbsp olive oil, salt and pepper.
3. Spread on lined baking sheet and roast for 25-30 minutes, until tender.
4. Combine lentils, sweet potato, and spinach.
5. Whisk together 1 tbsp olive oil, lemon juice, cumin, salt, and pepper in a small bowl and pour over salad.

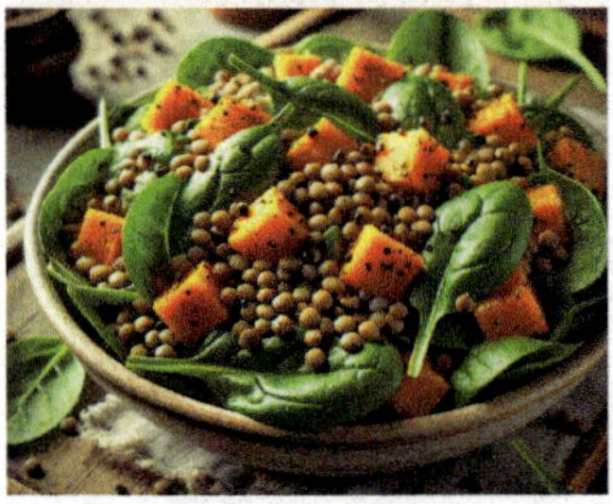

NUTRITION

- Calories: 350
- Macros: 14g fat, 45g carbs, 12g protein

This hearty salad is loaded with plant-based protein, fiber, and anti-inflammatory ingredients like olive oil and cumin.

Smoked Salmon and Avocado Wrap

INGREDIENTS

- 1 whole-grain wrap
- 2 oz smoked salmon
- ½ avocado, sliced
- 1 cup mixed greens
- 1 tbsp cream cheese (optional)
- 1 tsp lemon juice
- Salt and pepper to taste

DIRECTIONS

1. Spread cream cheese (if using) over the wrap and drizzle with lemon juice.
2. Layer with smoked salmon, avocado slices, and mixed greens.
3. Season with salt and pepper.
4. Roll the wrap tightly, cut in half, and serve.

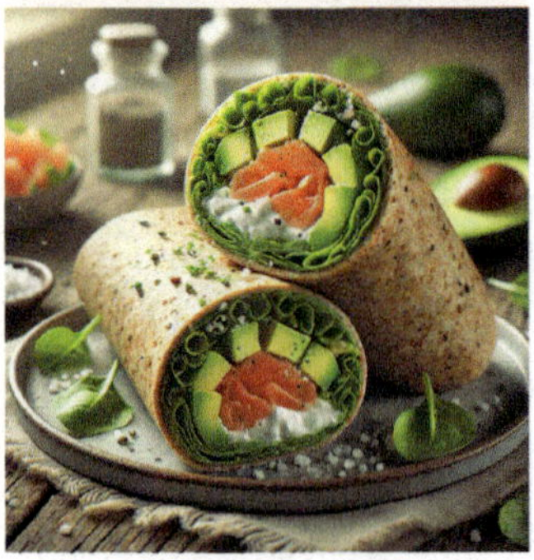

NUTRITION

- Calories: 340
- Macros: 18g fat, 30g carbs, 15g protein

This light yet satisfying wrap delivers omega-3 fatty acids and antioxidants for an anti-inflammatory boost.

Mediterranean Chickpea Salad

DIRECTIONS

1. Drain and rinse chickpeas.
2. Combine with cucumber, tomatoes, onion, and feta in a bowl.
3. Drizzle with olive oil and lemon juice.
4. Season with salt and pepper to taste

INGREDIENTS

- 8 oz canned chickpeas
- ½ cucumber, diced
- ¼ cup sliced tomatoes
- ¼ cup red onion, diced
- 2 tbsp feta cheese
- 1 tbsp olive oil
- 1 tbsp lemon juice
- Salt and pepper

NUTRITION

- Calories: 350
- Macros: 18g fat, 38g carbs, 12g protein

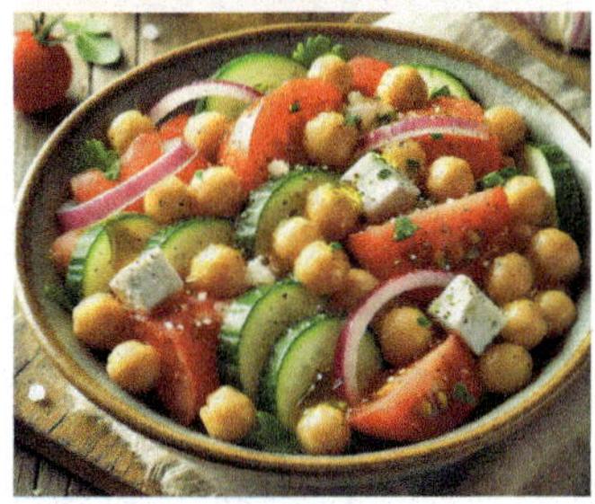

This salad is fresh and tasty, packed with fiber, healthy fats, and anti-inflammatory ingredients to nourish and satisfy.

Stuffed Bell Peppers

DIRECTIONS

1. Mix quinoa, black beans, corn, and cilantro. Season with salt and pepper.
2. Stuff the bell pepper halves with the above mixture.
3. Place in a baking dish, cover with foil, and bake at 375°F (190°C) for 20-30 minutes.

INGREDIENTS

- 2 bell peppers, with tops, seeds and membranes removed
- 1 cup cooked quinoa
- ½ cup black beans, drained and rinsed
- ¼ cup corn
- 1 tbsp fresh cilantro, chopped
- Salt and pepper

NUTRITION

- Calories: 380
- Macros: 8g fat, 65g carbs, 14g protein

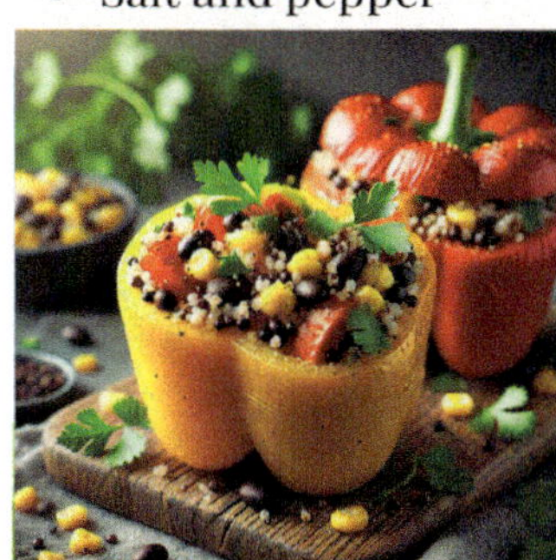

These Stuffed Bell Peppers are a colorful, nutrient-rich dish full of plant-based protein, fiber, and anti-inflammatory ingredients, making it a wholesome and satisfying meal.

Butternut Squash and Kale Salad with Tahini Dressing

INGREDIENTS

- 2 cups butternut squash, peeled and diced
- 2 cups kale, chopped
- 2 tbsp olive oil
- 2-3 tbsp Lemon Tahini dressing (see chapter 6)
- Salt and pepper

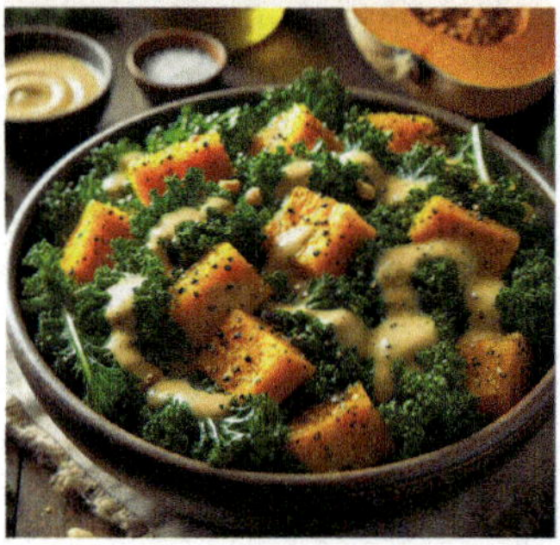

DIRECTIONS

1. Preheat oven to 400°F (200°C).
2. Toss butternut squash with 1 tbsp olive oil, salt, and pepper.
3. Roast for 25-30 minutes until tender.
4. In a large bowl, massage chopped kale with remaining olive oil and a pinch of salt until slightly wilted.
5. Combine roasted squash with kale and drizzle with tahini dressing. Toss to coat and serve.

NUTRITION

- Calories: 360
- Macros: 20g fat, 40g carbs, 6g protein

This vibrant salad is packed with fiber, antioxidants, and a creamy tahini dressing for anti-inflammatory benefits.

Cauliflower Rice Bowl with Tofu and Veggies

INGREDIENTS

- 1 block firm tofu
- 1 cup cauliflower rice
- 1 cup bell peppers, carrots, and broccoli
- 2 tbsp olive oil
- 1 tsp turmeric
- 1 tsp ginger, minced
- 1 tbsp low sodium soy sauce (optional - or coconut aminos if soy free)
- Salt and pepper

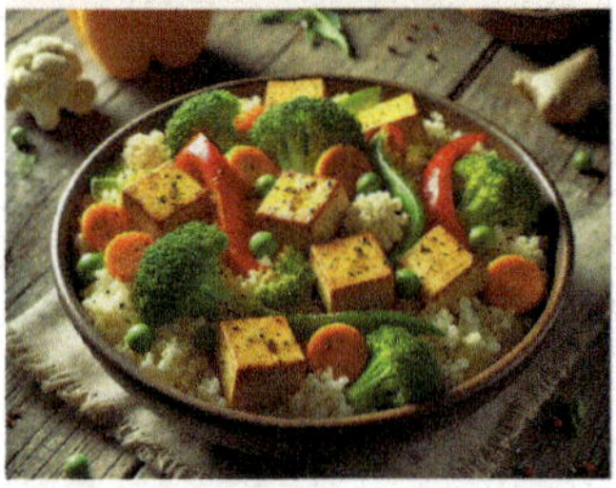

DIRECTIONS

1. Add cubed tofu to heated skillet with 1 tbsp olive oil.
2. Sauté until golden brown, about 5-7 minutes. Remove from pan.
3. In the same skillet, add remaining olive oil, vegetables, turmeric, and ginger.
4. Cook 4-5 minutes until tender.
5. Add cauliflower rice and cook 3-4 minutes.
6. Return tofu to skillet, toss with soy sauce (or coconut aminos if soy free),
7. Season with salt and pepper.

NUTRITION

- Calories: 330
- Macros: 22g fat, 18g carbs, 16g protein

A low-carb, plant-based bowl rich in anti-inflammatory compounds like turmeric and ginger.

Grilled Chicken and Quinoa Salad

DIRECTIONS

1. Season chicken with spice mixture.
2. Cook on grill or grill pan for 6-7 minutes per side or until fully cooked.
3. Let rest for 5 minutes, then slice.
4. Combine cooked quinoa, mixed greens, cucumber, and tomatoes, then top with chicken.
5. In a small bowl, whisk together olive oil, lemon juice, salt, and pepper.
6. Drizzle dressing over salad just before serving and toss to combine.

INGREDIENTS

- 1 chicken breast (6 oz)
- 1 tbsp anti-inflammatory spice mixture
- 1 cup cooked quinoa
- 2 cups mixed greens
- ¼ cup cucumber, sliced
- ¼ cup cherry tomatoes, halved
- 2 tbsp olive oil
- Juice of 1 lemon
- Salt and pepper

NUTRITION

- Calories: 450
- Macros: 20g fat, 40g carbs, 32g protein

Grilled chicken can be batch cooked and made ahead, to save time on busy mornings, when putting lunches together.

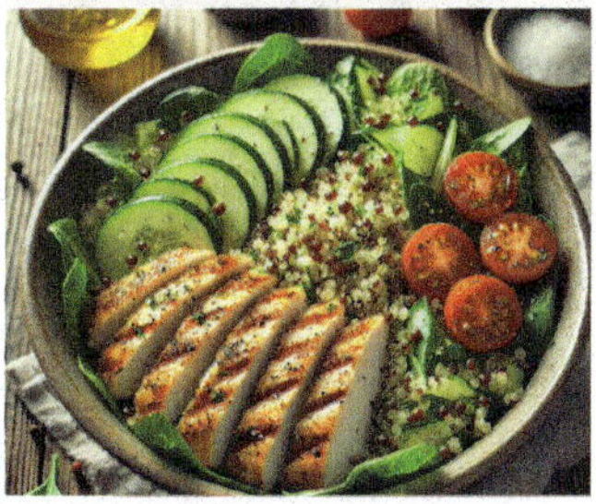

Turkey, Avocado, and Spinach Wrap

DIRECTIONS

1. Spread Dijon mustard evenly over the whole-grain wrap.
2. Layer with turkey breast slices, avocado, and spinach.
3. Sprinkle with salt and pepper.
4. Roll the wrap tightly and cut in half before serving.

INGREDIENTS

- 1 whole-grain wrap or tortilla
- 4 slices turkey breast
- ½ avocado, sliced
- 1 cup fresh spinach
- 1 tbsp Dijon mustard
- Salt and pepper to taste

NUTRITION

- Calories: 340
- Macros: 16g fat, 36g carbs, 20g protein

This easy and nutritious wrap provides a healthy dose of protein, fiber, and anti-inflammatory fats.

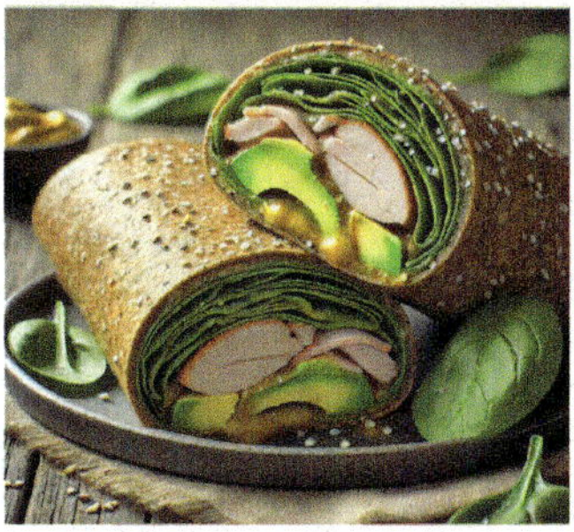

Roasted Beet and Arugula Salad with Goat Cheese

INGREDIENTS

- 2 medium beets
- 2 cups arugula
- ¼ cup goat cheese, crumbled
- 2-3 tbsp balsamic vinaigrette
- Salt and pepper to taste

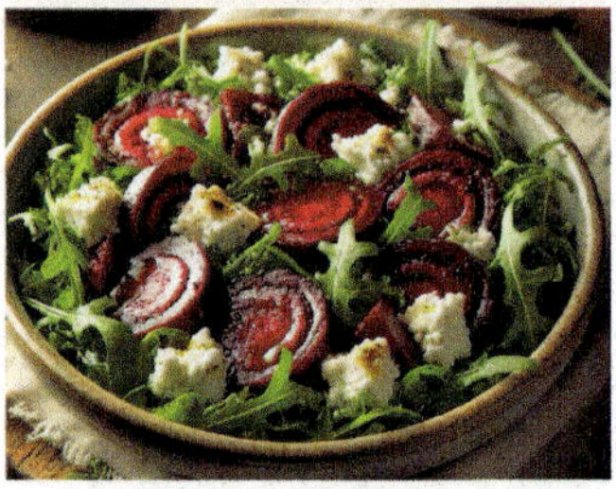

DIRECTIONS

1. Preheat oven to 400°F (200°C).
2. Wrap beets in foil and roast for 45-50 minutes, until tender.
3. Once cooled, peel and slice beets.
4. In a large bowl, toss arugula with balsamic vinaigrette dressing.
5. Top with roasted, sliced beets and goat cheese.

NUTRITION

- Calories: 300
- Macros: 21g fat, 21g carbs, 7g protein

This vibrant salad combines anti-inflammatory beets with the peppery flavor of arugula and creamy goat cheese.

Soba Noodle Salad with Edamame and Sesame Dressing

INGREDIENTS

- 4 oz soba noodles
- 1 cup shelled edamame (cooked)
- 1 carrot, shredded
- 1 tbsp sesame oil
- 2 tbsp soy sauce (or tamari if gluten-free)
- 1 tbsp rice vinegar
- 1 tsp fresh ginger, grated
- 1 tbsp sesame seeds

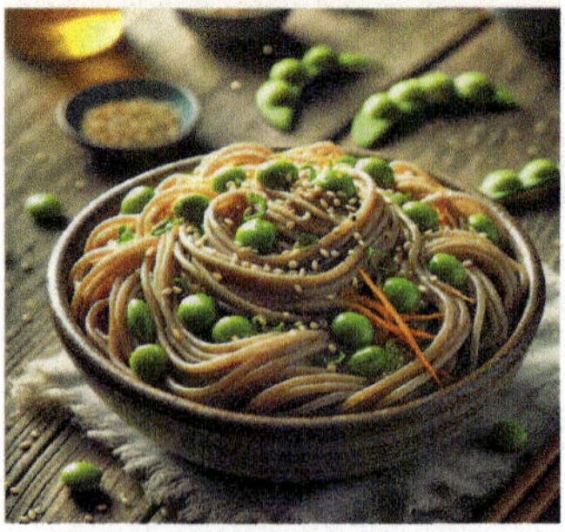

DIRECTIONS

1. Cook soba noodles according to package instructions. Drain and rinse under cold water.
2. In a small bowl, whisk together sesame oil, soy sauce, rice vinegar, and ginger.
3. In a large bowl, combine soba noodles, edamame, shredded carrot, and sesame seeds.
4. Pour the dressing over the noodle mixture and toss to combine.
5. Serve chilled or at room temperature.

NUTRITION

- Calories: 370
- Macros: 14g fat, 47g carbs, 14g protein

This light, Asian-inspired salad is packed with fiber and anti-inflammatory ingredients like ginger and sesame.

Roasted Tomato and Red Pepper Soup

DIRECTIONS

1. Preheat oven to 400°F (200°C).
2. Toss tomatoes, red peppers, and onion with olive oil, salt, and pepper. Place on a lined baking sheet and roast for 30-35 minutes or until tender.
3. Transfer to a blender, add other ingredients, and blend until smooth.
4. Pour soup into a pot, bring to a simmer, and cook for 5 minutes.
5. Serve hot, optionally with a slice of whole-grain bread.

INGREDIENTS

- 4 large tomatoes, halved
- 2 red bell peppers, halved and seeded
- 1 onion, chopped
- 2 cloves garlic, minced
- 2 cups vegetable broth
- 2 tbsp olive oil
- 1 tsp smoked paprika
- Salt and pepper

NUTRITION

- Calories: 280
- Macros: 18g fat, 28g carbs, 4g protein

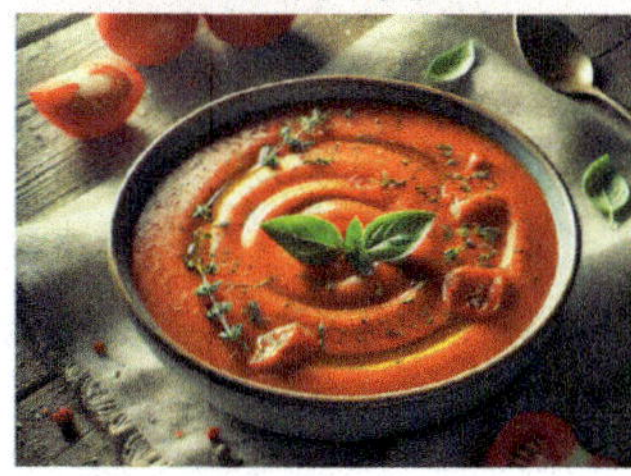

This comforting, antioxidant-rich dish fights inflammation with each spoonful.

Chicken and Avocado Lettuce Wraps

DIRECTIONS

1. Place the lettuce leaves on a plate or use them as wraps.
2. Add chicken, avocado slices, cucumber, and shredded carrots to each lettuce leaf.
3. Drizzle with olive oil and lime juice.
4. Sprinkle with salt and pepper.
5. Wrap the lettuce leaves around the fillings and serve.

INGREDIENTS

- 1 grilled chicken breast, sliced
- 1 avocado, sliced
- 6 large lettuce leaves
- ½ cucumber, sliced
- ½ cup shredded carrots
- 1 tbsp olive oil
- Juice of ½ lime
- Salt and pepper

NUTRITION

- Calories: 350
- Macros: 22g fat, 15g carbs, 25g protein

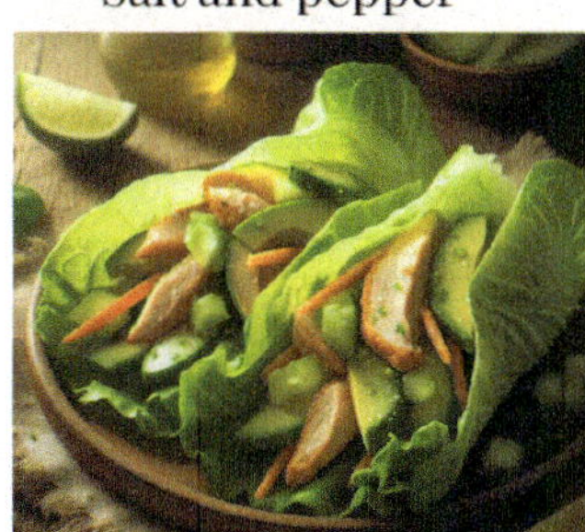

These easy-to-make lettuce wraps are perfect for a light, anti-inflammatory meal.

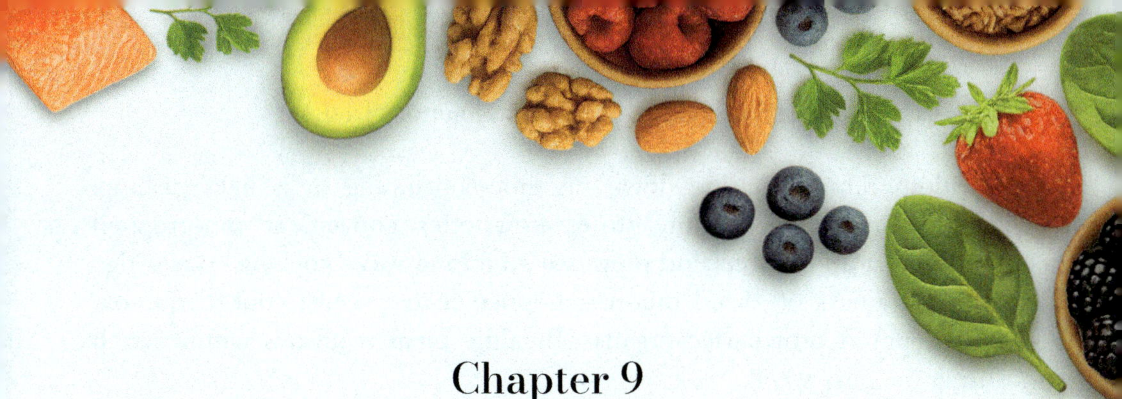

Chapter 9

Dinners to Calm Inflammation

Dinner, often a gathering point for families or a moment of solitary reflection, can be both a sanctuary and a battleground in the fight against chronic inflammation. With strategic approaches to meal preparation, it is possible to transform this pivotal meal into an ally for health.

In today's busy world, efficient cooking techniques are essential for maintaining a healthy, anti-inflammatory diet without sacrificing time. One-pan meals are perfect for this balance, offering convenience and health in one dish. Picture a sheet pan filled with salmon fillets nestled among vibrant vegetables like bell peppers, zucchini, and cherry tomatoes. These ingredients, drizzled with olive oil and herbs, combine their unique anti-inflammatory properties into a flavorful and nourishing meal with minimal prep and cleanup.

Pre-Prepped Ingredients

Saving time in the kitchen often starts with preparation. Pre-chopped vegetables and pre-cooked grains can serve as the building blocks for a nutritious dinner, cutting down on time-consuming tasks like washing, peeling, and dicing. Many stores now offer convenient pre-prepped options, but a little weekend prep can go a long way. Stocking your fridge with containers of diced onions, chopped leafy greens, cooked quinoa, and prepared brown rice means a healthy meal is always within reach during the busy week.

The idea that healthy meals require hours in the kitchen is a myth. With the right strategies, it's entirely possible to have dinner on the table in 30 minutes or less. Zucchini noodles tossed with a quick homemade pesto of basil, walnuts, and garlic provide a fresh, flavorful alternative to pasta, packed with anti-inflammatory benefits. Another fast favorite is chicken seasoned with anti-inflammatory spice mix, served over a bed of spinach and brown rice, blending the anti-inflammatory power of combined spices with the wholesomeness of whole grains and leafy greens—all within half an hour.

Simple Side Dishes

Side dishes can be more than just an afterthought—they can elevate a meal with their flavor and nutrients. Roasted Brussels sprouts, caramelized to crispy perfection, are loaded with fiber and antioxidants, while an arugula salad with strawberries, hemp seeds, and a light balsamic vinaigrette adds a refreshing contrast to heartier main dishes. Each side complements the main course while adding its own anti-inflammatory boost.

Simple, Easy Dinners

Even with just a few ingredients, you can create meals that are simple yet packed with flavor and nutrition. Take skillet-seared salmon, for example. Its crispy exterior pairs beautifully with a bed of wilted spinach, creating a dish rich in omega-3s and iron. This meal, topped with a drizzle of garlic-infused olive oil, becomes a weeknight staple that is satisfying and beneficial for your health.

One-pot meals shine in anti-inflammatory cooking, allowing flavors to meld together effortlessly. A stew made with turmeric, sweet potatoes, and lentils simmers away into a hearty, nourishing dish. As the turmeric adds anti-inflammatory properties, the sweet potatoes and lentils provide fiber and protein, making this meal comforting and healthful. With minimal prep required, this one-pot dish is a perfect blend of ease and wellness.

Anti-inflammatory Dinner Recipes

The dinner recipes included in this book bring both flavors and nutrients together. They are grounded in the powerful principles of anti-inflammatory eating. From vibrant vegetable-forward dishes to lean proteins paired with nourishing grains, each recipe is crafted to support your health, reduce inflammation, and enhance overall well-being.

Each dish serves as a reminder that food has the power to be both medicine and a source of enjoyment, capable of shaping our health with every bite. As you cook your way through these recipes, you may discover new favorite dishes that offer comfort, vitality, and satisfaction. These meals invite you to reconnect with the idea that cooking is both self-care and a means of nurturing the ones you love.

Sheet-Pan Salmon with Veggies

INGREDIENTS

- 2 - 6 oz salmon fillets
- 2 bell peppers, sliced
- 2 zucchinis, sliced
- 8 oz cherry tomatoes, halved
- 3 tbsp olive oil
- 2 cloves garlic
- Juice of ½ lemon
- 1 tsp oregano
- 1 tsp thyme
- Salt and pepper
- Lemon wedges and chopped parsley

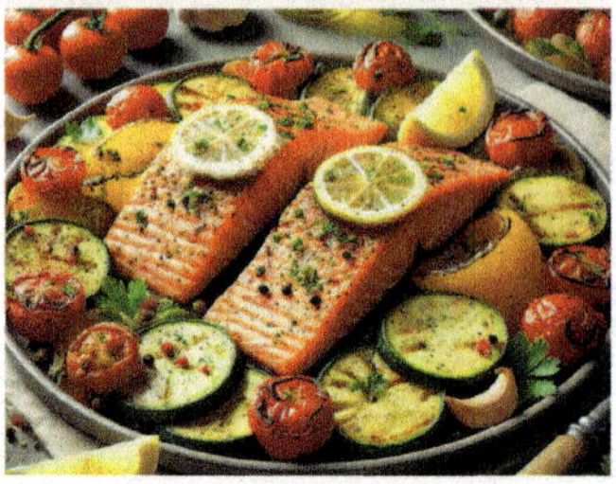

DIRECTIONS

1. Preheat oven to 400°F (200°C)
2. Toss veggies with 2 tbsp of olive oil, minced garlic, oregano, thyme, salt, and pepper.
3. Place veggies and salmon fillets on a sheet pan lined with parchment paper.
4. Drizzle filllets with 1 tbsp olive oil and lemon juice; season with salt pepper.
5. Roast 15-18 minutes, or until salmon flakes easily with a fork and the vegetables are tender.
6. Garnish with parsley and serve with lemon wedges.

NUTRITION

- Calories (per serving): 400
- Macros: 25g fat, 15g carbs, 32g protein

This sheet-pan meal features omega-3-rich salmon and vibrant, anti-inflammatory vegetables.

Grilled Chicken with Sautéed Spinach and Brown Rice

INGREDIENTS

- 2 chicken breasts (6oz)
- 1 tbsp olive oil
- 2 cups spinach
- 1 garlic clove
- ½ cup cooked brown rice
- 1 tbsp Anti-inflammatory spice
- Salt and pepper
- 2 tbsp Creamy Mango Dressing (chapter 6)

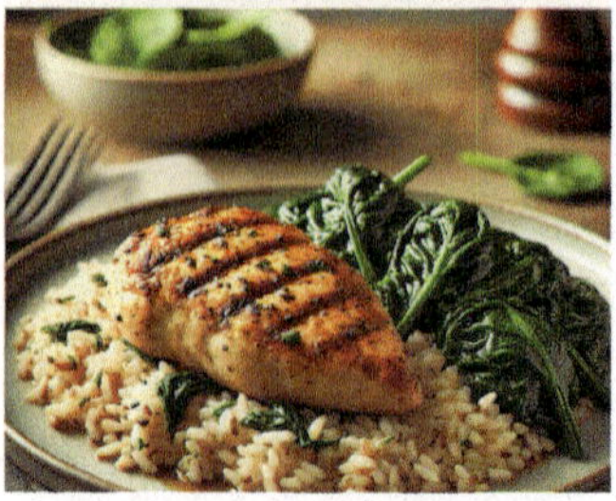

DIRECTIONS

1. Season chicken with spice mixture, salt, and pepper.
2. Grill chicken over medium heat on grill or grill pan 6-7 minutes per side or until fully cooked.
3. Sauté minced garlic in olive oil for 1 minute, then add spinach and cook 2-3 minutes, until wilted.
4. Season with a pinch of salt and pepper.
5. Serve chicken over cooked brown rice with sautéed spinach on the side and Creamy Mango Dressing for dipping.

NUTRITION

- Calories: 500
- Macros: 20g fat, 42g carbs, 42g protein

This simple and nutritious meal is a balanced, anti-inflammatory dish rich in protein, fiber, and healthy fats.

Stir-Fried Tofu with Vegetables over Quinoa

DIRECTIONS

1. Add cubed tofu to heated skillet with ½ tbsp olive oil and sauté until golden on all sides, about 5-6 minutes.
2. Remove from pan and set aside.
3. Add ½ tbsp olive oil, ginger, and turmeric to pan. Sauté for 1 minute.
4. Add vegetables and cook for 5-7 minutes, stirring occasionally, until tender-crisp.
5. Return tofu to pan. Add lemon juice, salt, and pepper to taste; toss to combine.
6. Serve over a bed of cooked quinoa.

INGREDIENTS

- ½ block tofu, cubed
- 1 tbsp olive oil
- 1 cup mixed veggies (broccoli, bell peppers, snap peas)
- 1 tsp grated ginger
- ¼ tsp turmeric
- Juice of ½ lemon
- Salt and pepper
- 1 cup cooked quinoa

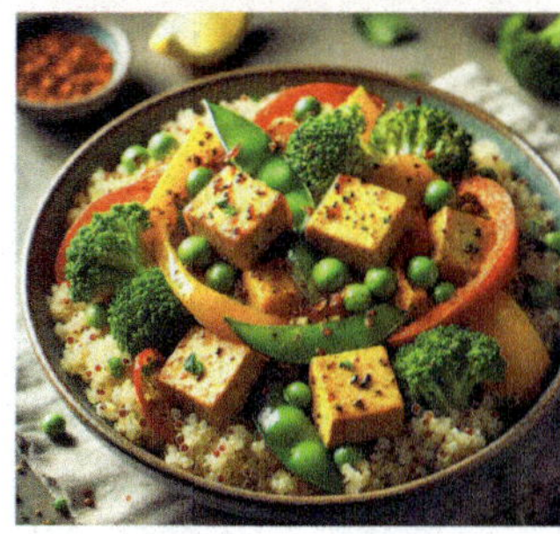

NUTRITION

- Calories: 450
- Macros: 23g fat, 45g carbs, 20g protein

You may swap tofu for other lean proteins if you desire.

Turkey Chili

DIRECTIONS

1. In a large pot, cook ground turkey, garlic, and onion until meat is browned and onion is softened.
2. Drain and rinse kidney beans and add to pot, along with other ingredients.
3. Bring the mixture to a simmer, reduce heat to low, cover, and cook for 20 minutes, stirring occasionally, until slightly thickened.
4. Taste and adjust seasoning if needed.

INGREDIENTS

- 1 lb ground turkey
- 1 cup kidney beans
- 1 bell pepper, diced
- 1 cup diced tomatoes
- 1 cup low-sodium chicken or vegetable broth
- 1 tsp chili powder
- 1 tsp cumin
- Salt and pepper
- 1 garlic clove, minced
- 1 small onion, diced

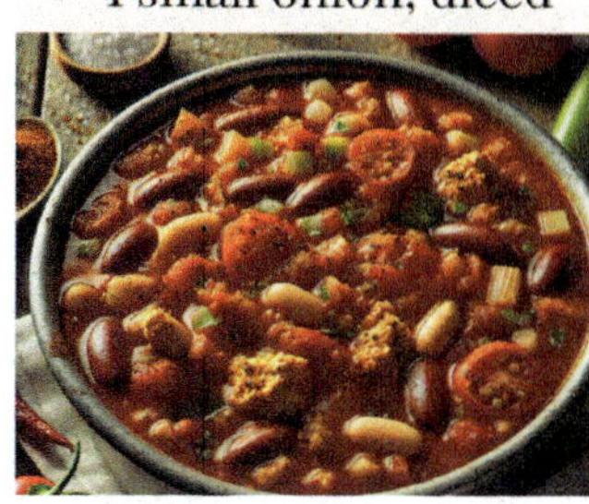

NUTRITION

- Calories: 450
- Macros: 16g fat, 45g carbs, 35g protein

This hearty chili is protein-packed and perfect for a cozy, healthy dinner that's both satisfying and easy to make.

Baked Cod with Roasted Brussels Sprouts and Quinoa

INGREDIENTS

- 2 cod fillets (6 oz)
- 1 cup Brussels sprouts, halved
- 1 tbsp olive oil
- 1 cup cooked quinoa
- Salt and pepper to taste
- Juice of ½ lemon
- Fresh parsley and lemon wedges for garnish (optional)

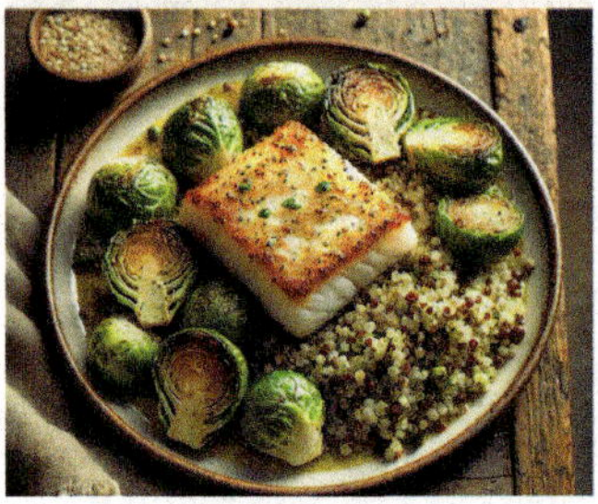

DIRECTIONS

1. Preheat oven to 400°F (200°C).
2. Toss Brussels sprouts with ½ tbsp olive oil. Add a pinch of salt and pepper.
3. Roast 20-25 minutes on lined baking sheet until golden with crispy edges.
4. Prepare cod with ½ tbsp olive oil, lemon juice, salt and pepper.
5. Bake with Brussels sprouts for the last 12-15 minutes.
6. Cook quinoa according to package instructions.
7. Garnish with fresh parsley and lemon.

NUTRITION

- Calories: 450
- Macros: 18g fat, 40g carbs, 40g protein

This easy and nutritious meal offers a delicious combination of textures and flavors to keep you feeling satisfied.

Zucchini Noodles with Pesto and Cherry Tomatoes

INGREDIENTS

- 2 large zucchinis
- 1 cup cherry tomatoes, halved
- 1 tbsp olive oil
- 2 tbsp basil walnut pesto (chapter 6)
- Salt and pepper
- Fresh basil and grated Parmesan cheese for garnish

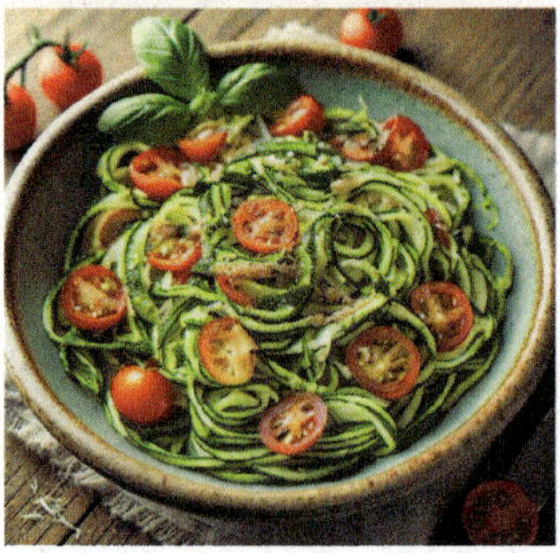

DIRECTIONS

1. Use a spiralizer or julienne peeler to create zucchini noodles.
2. Sauté "noodles" in large skillet with olive oil for 3-5 minutes until slightly tender. Avoid overcooking.
3. Add cherry tomatoes and cook for another minute.
4. Add pesto and toss to evenly coat.
5. Season with salt and pepper to taste.
6. Serve with fresh basil and Parmesan if desired.

NUTRITION

- Calories: 350
- Macros: 28g fat, 18g carbs, 8g protein

Add sliced chicken breast or chopped nuts for added protein, and other veggies like roasted red peppers for variety.

Baked Chicken Breasts with Root Vegetables and Brown Rice

DIRECTIONS

1. Preheat oven to 400°F (200°C).
2. Place chicken breasts and vegetables on lined baking sheet.
3. Drizzle with olive oil and season with salt and pepper.
4. Bake for 25-30 minutes, or until chicken is done and vegetables are tender and lightly browned.
5. Prepare brown rice as directed.
6. Garnish with fresh herbs and lemon wedges.

INGREDIENTS

- 2 chicken breasts
- 1 cup carrots (and parsnips, if desired)
- 1 tbsp olive oil
- 1 cup cooked brown rice
- Salt and pepper, to taste
- Fresh thyme or rosemary for garnish
- Lemon wedges

NUTRITION

- Calories: 500
- Macros: 22g fat, 45g carbs, 35g protein

This simple yet satisfying meal provides lean protein, complex carbohydrates, and plenty of nutrients to keep you fueled and feeling full.

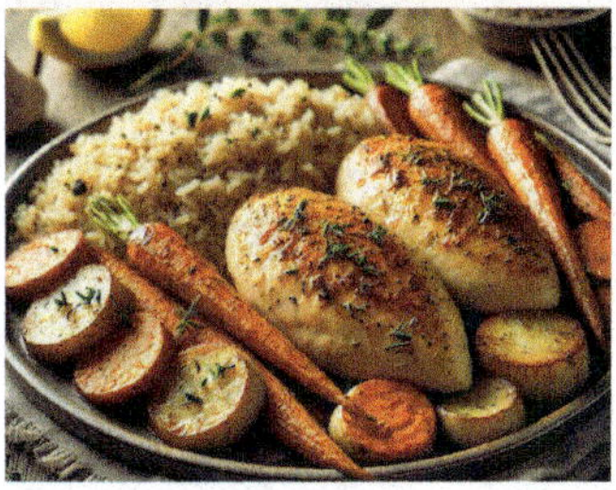

Spicy Beef and Veggie Stir-Fry

DIRECTIONS

1. Chop veggies and thinly slice beef against the grain.
2. Salt and pepper beef. In wok or skillet, stir-fry with oil until browned but slightly pink in the center. Remove from skillet.
3. Add more oil and season veggies with salt and chili flakes.
4. Stir-fry 3-4 minutes til tender-crisp.
5. Return beef to skillet and stir-fry for 1-2 minutes, until cooked through.
6. Add soy sauce or coconut aminos.
7. Serve over brown rice and garnish with green onions or sesame seeds.

INGREDIENTS

- 4 oz lean beef
- 8 oz bell pepper, zucchini, snap peas
- 1-2 tbsps olive or sesame oil
- 1 tsp chili flakes
- Salt and pepper
- 8 oz cooked brown rice
- Low sodium soy sauce or coconut aminos if soy-free
- Chopped green onion

NUTRITION

- Calories: 400
- Macros: 20g fat, 50g carbs, 30g protein

This quick and flavorful stir-fry combines lean beef with fresh, colorful vegetables and a hint of spice.

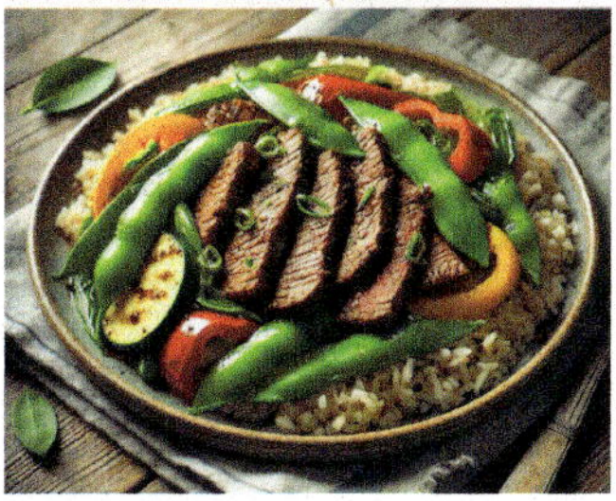

Grilled Salmon with Asparagus and Turmeric-Spiced Quinoa

INGREDIENTS

- 2 salmon fillets (6 oz)
- 8 oz asparagus
- 1 tbsp olive oil, divided
- 1 cup cooked quinoa
- 1 tsp ground turmeric
- Salt and pepper
- Lemon wedges and fresh parsley for garnish

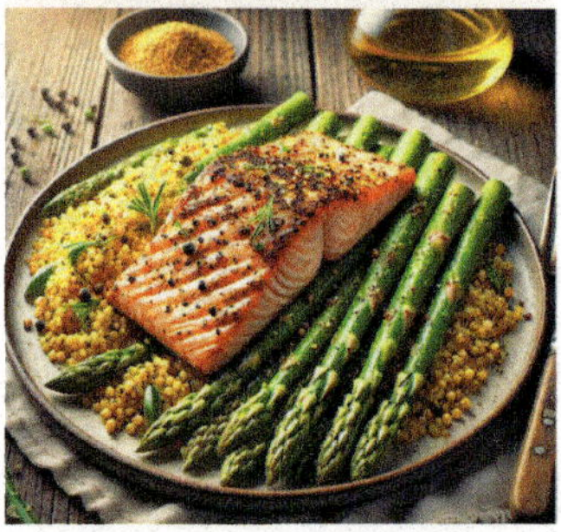

DIRECTIONS

1. Salt and pepper salmon fillets.
2. Cook on oiled grill or grill pan for 4-5 minutes on each side or until salmon flakes easily with a fork.
3. Add asparagus to a skillet with ½ tbsp of olive oil, salt, and pepper, and sauté until tender-crisp.
4. In a separate bowl, toss warm, cooked quinoa with turmeric and remaining olive oil until evenly coated. Salt and pepper to taste.
5. Serve with fresh lemon wedges and a sprinkle of fresh parsley, if desired.

NUTRITION

- Calories: 500
- Macros: 26g fat, 32g carbs, 38g protein

This meal has protein, fiber, healthy fats, and the antioxidant properties of turmeric.

Chicken and Vegetable Skewers with Brown Rice and Tzatziki

INGREDIENTS

- 1 chicken breast, cubed
- 1 cup bell peppers, zucchini, and onions
- 1 tbsp olive oil
- Salt and pepper
- 8 oz cooked brown rice
- ¼ cup tzatziki (ch. 6)
- Lemon wedges
- Fresh parsley or dill

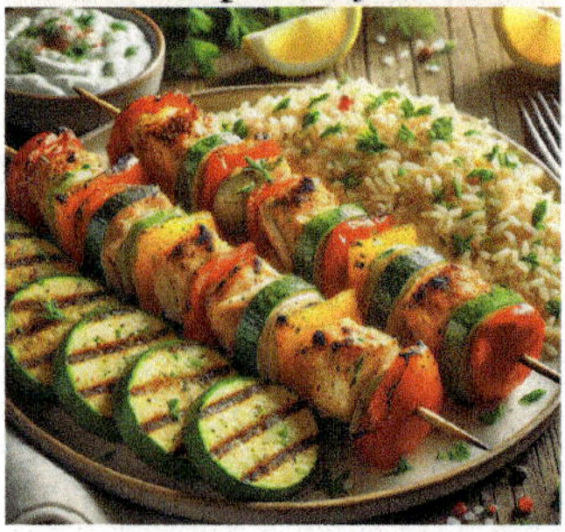

DIRECTIONS

1. Soak wooden skewers in water 15-20 minutes. Alternate chicken and vegetable pieces on skewers. Brush with olive oil. Salt and pepper.
2. Place skewers on heated grill or grill pan and cook 10-12 minutes, turning occasionally, until chicken is cooked and vegetables are tender.
3. Cook brown rice according to package directions.
4. Serve skewers over brown rice with a side of tzatziki. Garnish with lemon wedges and fresh parsley or dill.

NUTRITION

- Calories: 480
- Macros: 20g fat, 45g carbs, 35g protein

Rich in protein, fiber, and essential nutrients, this dish is perfect for a satisfying and wholesome dinner.

Baked Eggplant Parmesan with Mixed Greens Salad

DIRECTIONS

1. Preheat oven to 375°F (190°C) .
2. Layer ¼-inch eggplant rounds in an oiled baking dish.
3. Top with marinara and Parmesan.
4. Repeat layers, finishing with a final sprinkle of Parmesan on top.
5. Cover with foil; bake 15 minutes, then uncover and bake 10 minutes more.
6. Garnish with fresh basil or parsley.
7. Toss mixed greens with balsamic vinaigrette.

INGREDIENTS

- 1 medium eggplant
- ½ cup marinara sauce (chapter 6)
- ¼ cup grated Parmesan
- 1 tsp olive oil
- 2 cups mixed greens
- 2 tbsp balsamic vinaigrette
- Salt and pepper
- Fresh basil or parsley

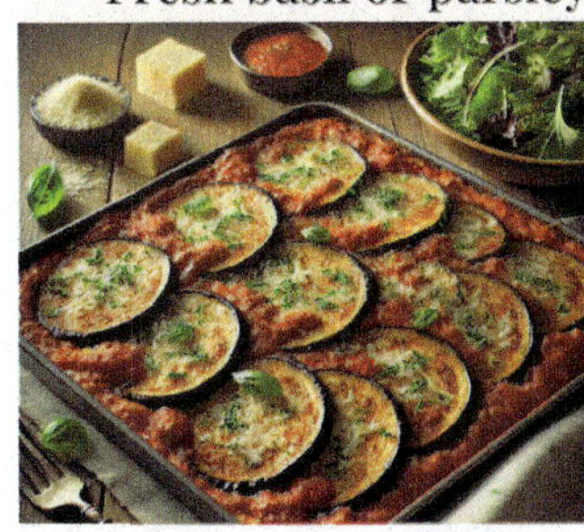

NUTRITION

- Calories: 450
- Macros: 22g fat, 45g carbs, 18g protein

This balanced meal combines comforting flavors with nutritious ingredients, perfect for a wholesome, Italian-inspired dinner.

Spiced Chicken with Roasted Cauliflower and Carrot Fries

DIRECTIONS

1. Preheat oven to 375°F (190°C).
2. Rub chicken breasts with 1 tbsp olive oil and anti-inflammatory spice mix.
3. Toss vegetables with 1 tbsp olive oil; sprinkle with salt and pepper.
4. Put chicken breasts, cauliflower, and carrots on lined baking sheet.
5. Bake for 25-30 minutes, or until chicken is done and vegetables are tender and golden.
6. Slice chicken and plate with veggies.

INGREDIENTS

- 2 chicken breasts
- Anti-inflammatory spice mix
- 1 cup cauliflower florets
- 2 medium carrots, peeled and cut into fries
- 2 tbsp olive oil
- Salt and pepper

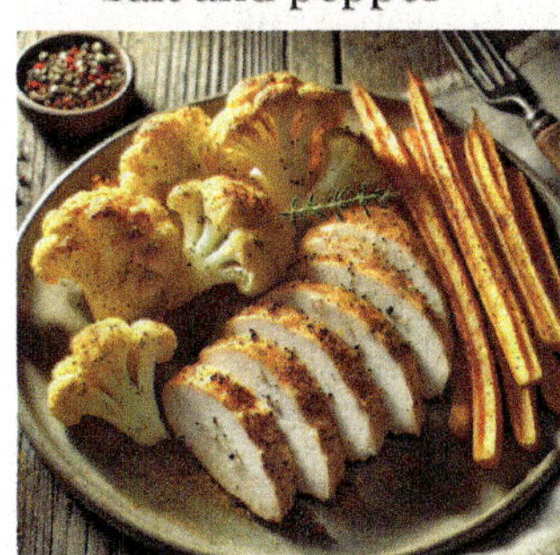

NUTRITION

- Calories: 350
- Macros: 14g fat, 45g carbs, 12g protein

This deliciously seasoned chicken pairs perfectly with roasted cauliflower and carrot fries for a nutrient-rich meal.

Shrimp Stir-Fry with Broccoli, Snap Peas, and Brown Rice

INGREDIENTS

- 8-10 medium shrimp
- 1 cup broccoli florets
- 1 cup snap peas
- 1 tbsp olive oil
- 1 tbsp low-sodium soy sauce
- 1 tsp fresh ginger
- 8 oz cooked brown rice
- Salt and pepper
- Sesame seeds
- Fresh lime

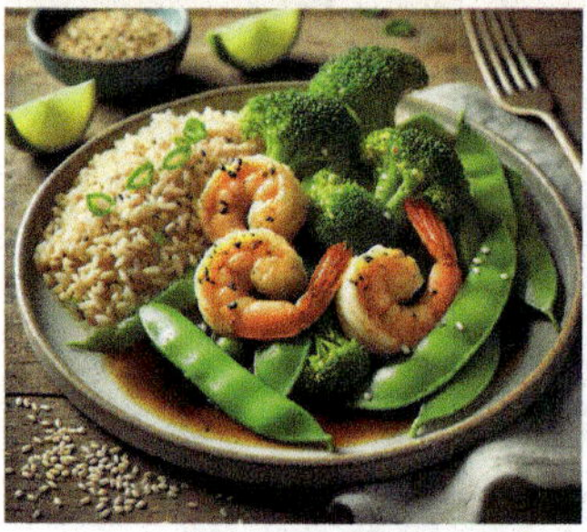

DIRECTIONS

1. Peel and devein shrimp, lightly salt and pepper, and add to olive oil in heated wok or skillet.
2. Sauté 2-3 minutes or until shrimp turn pink and are cooked through.
3. Remove from pan.
4. Stir-fry veggies and minced ginger for 4-5 minutes or until tender-crisp.
5. Add soy sauce and toss to coat.
6. Return shrimp to pan and continue cooking for 1-2 minutes.
7. Serve with cooked brown rice.
8. Garnish with sesame seeds and lime.

NUTRITION

- Calories: 450
- Macros: 16g fat, 50g carbs, 30g protein

This quick, nutrient-dense meal is a flavorful and satisfying choice for dinner.

Pesto Chicken with Roasted Asparagus

INGREDIENTS

- 2 chicken breasts
- 4 tbsp basil walnut pesto (chapter 6)
- 1 cup asparagus
- 2 tbsp olive oil
- Salt and pepper
- Basil and Parmesan for garnish
- Lemon wedge

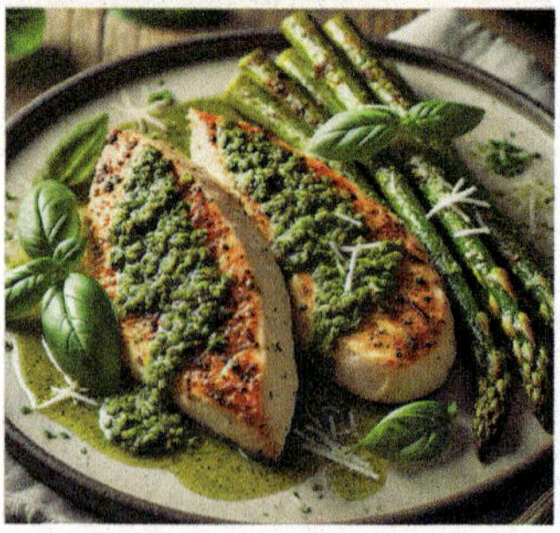

DIRECTIONS

1. Preheat oven to 400°F (200°C).
2. Lightly salt and pepper chicken.
3. Spread each with 1 tbsp of pesto.
4. Drizzle asparagus with olive oil, season with salt and pepper, and toss to coat.
5. Place chicken and asparagus on lined baking sheet.
6. Bake 20-25 minutes, or until chicken is done. Remove asparagus after 15 minutes, or when tender.
7. Garnish with extra pesto, fresh basil, Parmesan, and lemon.

NUTRITION

- Calories: 480
- Macros: 24g fat, 10g carbs, 35g protein

This simple yet flavorful dish requires minimal ingredients and prep.

Honey-Ginger Salmon with Steamed Broccoli

DIRECTIONS

1. Preheat your oven to 400°F (200°C).
2. Mix honey, grated ginger, and olive oil.
3. Salt and pepper salmon, then brush the top with honey-ginger glaze.
4. Bake 12-15 minutes on lined baking sheet, or until salmon flakes easily.
5. Steam broccoli in a steamer basket over boiling water for 5-7 minutes or until bright green and tender-crisp. Season with a pinch of salt.
6. May add more glaze before serving.
7. Garnish with sesame seeds and lemon wedges.

NUTRITION

- Calories: 450
- Macros: 20g fat, 25g carbs, 35g protein

This omega-3-rich meal has a delightful blend of sweetness and spice.

INGREDIENTS

- 1 salmon fillet (6 oz)
- 1 tbsp honey
- 1 tsp fresh ginger
- 1 tbsp olive oil
- 1 cup broccoli florets
- Salt and pepper
- Fresh lemon wedges, and sesame seeds for garnish

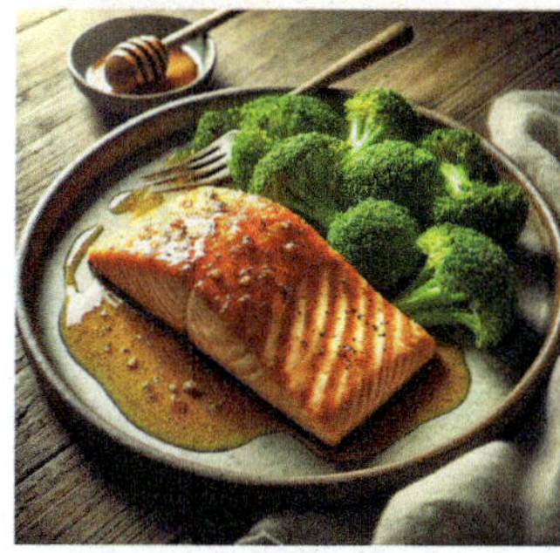

Rosemary and Garlic Pork Chops with Mashed Cauliflower

DIRECTIONS

1. Mix herbs, salt, and pepper and rub over pork chops. Let stand 5 minutes.
2. Sear meat in a hot skillet with 1 tbsp olive oil for 3-4 minutes on each side.
3. Remove from heat once internal temperature reaches 145°F (63°C), and let rest for 5 minutes.
4. Steam cauliflower for 8-10 minutes in a steamer basket over a pot of boiling water until fork-tender.
5. Add 1 tbsp olive oil, salt, and pepper and mash until smooth.
6. Garnish with parsley and lemon.

NUTRITION

- Calories: 450
- Macros: 30g fat, 12g carbs, 30g protein

Juicy pork chops and creamy mashed cauliflower are paired for a comforting, low-carb dinner.

INGREDIENTS

- 2 pork chops (6 oz)
- 2 tsp fresh rosemary (or 1 tsp dried)
- 2 cloves garlic
- Salt and pepper
- 2 tbsp olive oil, divided
- 2 cups cauliflower florets
- Fresh parsley
- Lemon wedges

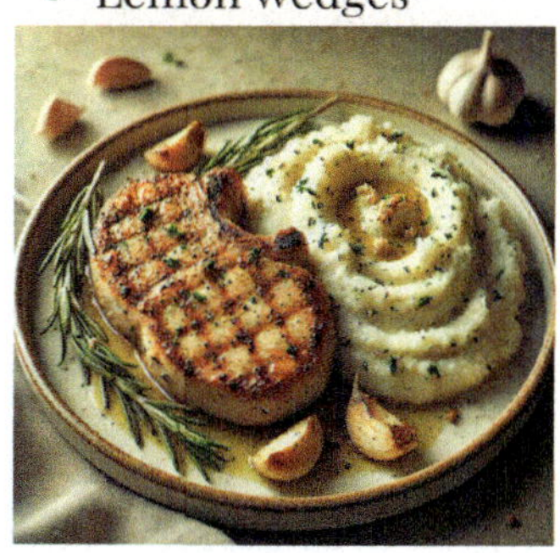

Lemon Herb Grilled Chicken with Roasted Sweet Potatoes

INGREDIENTS

- 2 chicken breasts
- 3 tbsp olive oil
- Juice of ½ lemon
- 1 tsp rosemary
- 1 tsp thyme,
- 1 cup sweet potato, diced into ½-inch cubes
- Salt and pepper
- Lemon slices

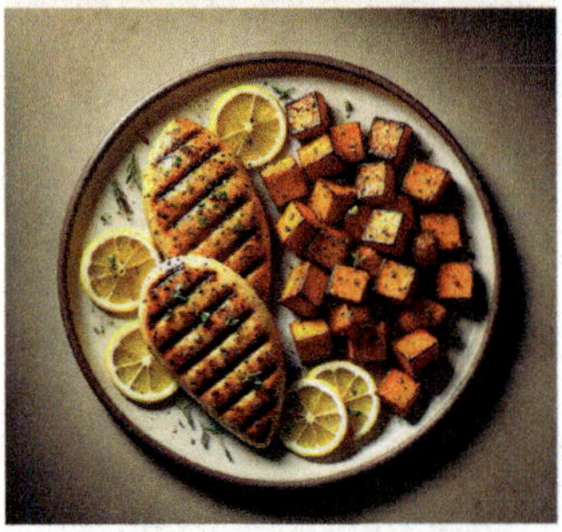

DIRECTIONS

1. Marinate chicken for ½ hour in 2 tbsp olive oil, lemon juice, dried herbs, salt, and pepper.
2. Preheat oven to 400°F (200°C).
3. Toss sweet potatoes with remaining olive oil, salt, and pepper on lined baking sheet.
4. Roast 20-25 minutes, or until tender.
5. Grill chicken on oiled grill or grill pan 6-7 minutes per side, or until done, then let rest 5 minutes before serving.

NUTRITION

- Calories: 400
- Macros: 16g fat, 35g carbs, 30g protein

This dish makes a wholesome, flavorful meal, perfect for any season.

Coconut Curry Lentil Soup

INGREDIENTS

- 1 tbsp coconut oil
- 1 onion, diced
- 2 cloves garlic
- 1 tbsp curry powder
- 1 cup red lentils
- 14 oz can coconut milk
- 24 oz vegetable broth
- Salt and pepper
- Fresh cilantro, lime wedges, or red chili flakes (optional)

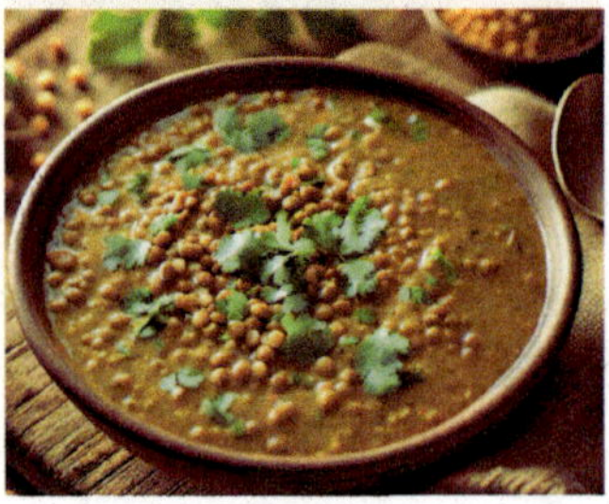

DIRECTIONS

1. Rinse lentils in fine mesh strainer.
2. Add coconut oil and onion to medium pan and sauté until softened.
3. Add garlic and sauté 1-2 minutes more.
4. Stir in curry powder and cook for 1 minute.
5. Add lentils, coconut milk, and broth.
6. Cover and simmer 20-25 minutes, until lentils soften and begin to break down slightly, then salt and pepper to taste.
7. If too thick, add more broth or water.
8. Serve with fresh cilantro, lime wedges, or red chili flakes for a little extra heat.

NUTRITION

- Calories: 480
- Macros: 26g fat, 45g carbs, 15g protein

This hearty soup is a satisfying dish, perfect for cozy dinners or meal prep.

Stuffed Bell Peppers with Quinoa and Turkey

DIRECTIONS

1. Preheat oven to 375°F (190°C).
2. Cook ground turkey in a large skillet, breaking it up as it cooks.
3. Add paprika, salt, and pepper and cook for another 1-2 minutes.
4. Add prepared quinoa and tomato sauce; cook for 2-3 minutes more.
5. Spoon turkey mixture into peppers, then place in oiled baking dish.
6. Cover with foil and bake 25-30 minutes until peppers are tender and filling is heated through.
7. Garnish with fresh parsley or basil.

INGREDIENTS

- 4 bell peppers (tops, seeds, and membranes removed)
- 1 tbsp olive oil
- 1 cup cooked quinoa
- ½ lb ground turkey
- 1 tsp smoked paprika
- Salt and pepper, to taste
- ½ cup tomato sauce
- Fresh parsley or basil

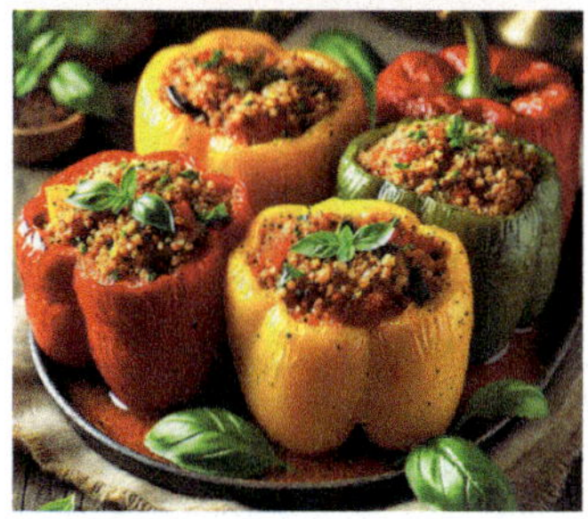

NUTRITION

- Calories: 500
- Macros: 22g fat, 45g carbs, 35g protein

These colorful stuffed bell peppers are a flavorful and nutritious meal.

Roasted Cod with Lemon and Thyme

DIRECTIONS

1. Preheat oven to 400°F (200°C).
2. Toss veggies with 1 tbsp of olive oil, salt, and pepper.
3. Drizzle cod fillets with 1 tbsp olive oil, lemon juice, thyme, salt, and pepper.
4. Place veggies and cod fillets on a lined baking sheet.
5. Roast for 12-15 minutes, or until fillets are opaque and flakes easily with a fork, and the vegetables are tender and lightly caramelized.
6. Serve with additional lemon wedges.

INGREDIENTS

- 2 cod fillets (6 oz)
- 2 tbsp olive oil
- Juice of ½ lemon
- 1 tsp fresh thyme (or ½ tsp dried thyme)
- Salt and pepper
- 1 cup zucchini, carrots, and cherry tomatoes (halved)
- Lemon wedges

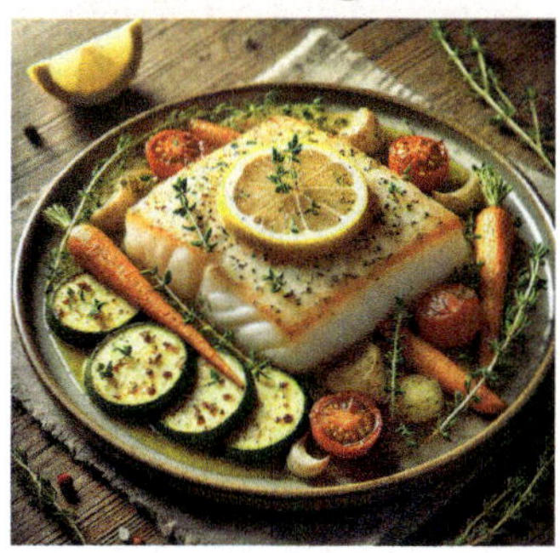

NUTRITION

- Calories: 350
- Macros: 20g fat, 10g carbs, 30g protein

This roasted cod is flavored with lemon and thyme, paired with a side of roasted veggies for a fresh and flavorful meal.

Chili Lime Shrimp Tacos with Shredded Cabbage

INGREDIENTS

- 1 cup shrimp
- 1 tsp chili powder
- Juice of 1 lime
- 1 tbsp olive oil
- 4 small corn tortillas
- 1 cup shredded cabbage
- Salt and pepper
- Cilantro and lime wedges
- 4 tbsp cilantro lime sauce (chapter 6)

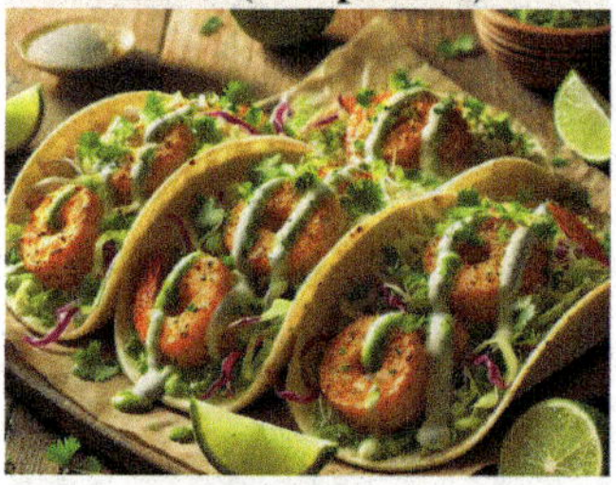

DIRECTIONS

1. Peel and devein shrimp
2. Toss shrimp with chili powder, lime juice, olive oil, salt, and pepper.
3. Transfer to a skillet and cook shrimp until pink.
4. Warm tortillas in a dry skillet about 30 seconds on each side.
5. Fill tortillas with shrimp and shredded cabbage.
6. Serve with cilantro lime sauce, fresh cilantro, and lime wedges.

NUTRITION

- Calories: 400
- Macros: 18g fat, 40g carbs, 25g protein

These zesty chili lime shrimp tacos with fresh cabbage are a light, flavorful dinner.

Moroccan-Spiced Lamb Chops with Roasted Vegetables

INGREDIENTS

- 2 lamb chops (6 oz)
- 1 tsp cumin
- 1 tsp coriander
- 1 tbsp olive oil
- 1 cup zucchini, bell peppers, and cherry tomatoes
- Salt and pepper
- Fresh parsley or dill
- Lemon wedges

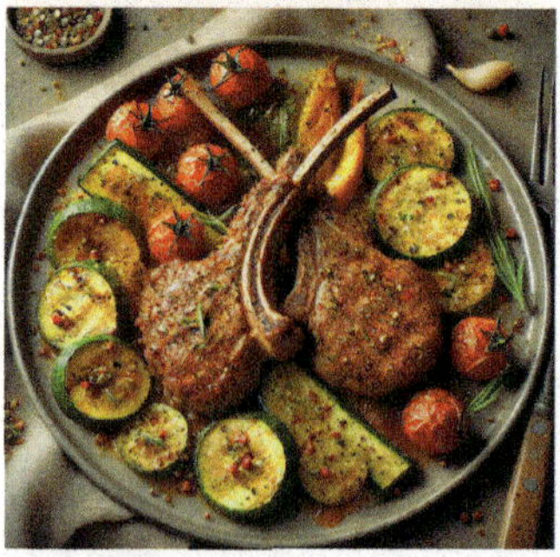

DIRECTIONS

1. Preheat oven to 400°F (200°C).
2. Drizzle lamb chops with ½ tbsp olive oil and rub in spices, salt, and pepper.
3. Toss veggies with ½ tbsp olive oil, salt, and pepper. Place on lined baking sheet with pork chops.
4. Roast 25 minutes, or until lamb reaches desired level of doneness and veggies are tender.
5. Rest chops 5 minutes before serving.
6. Garnish with fresh parsley or dill and serve with lemon wedges.

NUTRITION

- Calories: 480
- Macros: 35g fat, 15g carbs, 30g protein

For extra Moroccan flavor, sprinkle a pinch of cinnamon or smoked paprika over lamb chops before roasting.

Coconut Curry Chicken with Spinach and Brown Rice

DIRECTIONS

1. Cube, then salt and pepper chicken.
2. In a large pan, brown on all sides in coconut oil (about 4-5 minutes).
3. Sprinkle in curry powder, stir well, and cook 1-2 minutes more.
4. Add coconut milk and stir to combine.
5. Simmer 10-15 minutes until sauce thickens slightly.
6. Add spinach and cook for 2-3 minutes.
7. Serve curry over cooked brown rice.
8. Garnish with fresh cilantro or basil, and lime wedges.

INGREDIENTS

- 2 chicken breasts
- 1-2 tbsp coconut oil
- 1 tsp curry powder
- 1 cup coconut milk
- 2 cups fresh spinach, roughly chopped
- Salt and pepper
- 1 cup cooked brown rice
- Cilantro or basil
- Lime wedges

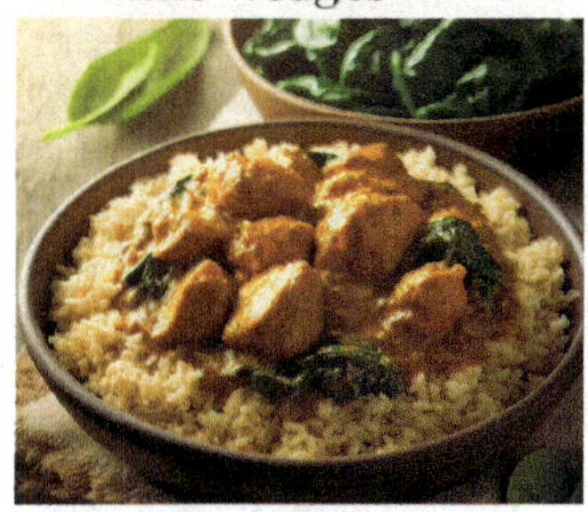

NUTRITION

- Calories: 450
- Macros: 32g fat, 8g carbs, 30g protein

This dish blends warming spices, rich coconut milk, and tender chicken.

Lemon-Garlic Chicken with Roasted Vegetables

DIRECTIONS

1. Preheat oven to 400°F (200°C).
2. Mix 1 tbsp olive oil, garlic, and lemon juice.
3. Rub mixture over chicken breasts.
4. Place chicken and vegetables on lined baking sheet.
5. Drizzle remaining olive oil over vegetables and season with salt and pepper.
6. Roast for 20-25 minutes until chicken is cooked and vegetables are tender.

INGREDIENTS

- 2 chicken breasts
- 2 tbsp olive oil
- 2 cloves garlic, minced
- Juice of ½ lemon
- Salt and pepper
- 1 cup carrots, zucchini, bell pepper (or your choice)

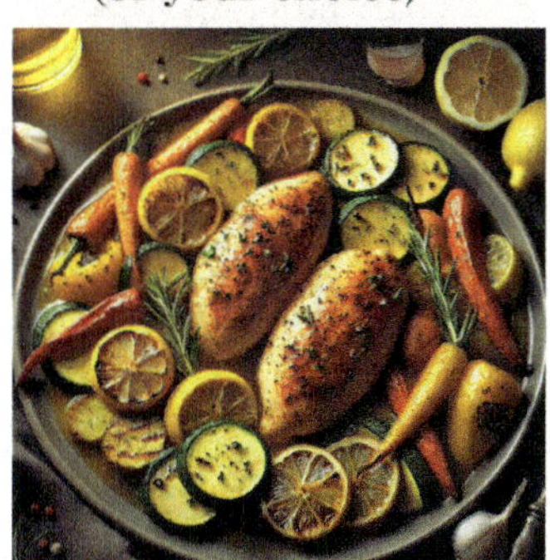

NUTRITION

- Calories: 400
- Macros: 22g fat, 20g carbs, 30g protein

This tangy lemon-garlic chicken with roasted vegetables is a flavorful, balanced meal that's easy to make.

Roasted Pork Tenderloin with Apple and Sweet Potato

INGREDIENTS

- 1 pork tenderloin (8 oz)
- 1 tbsp olive oil
- 1 tbsp anti-inflammatory spice
- 1 medium apple
- 1 sweet potato
- 1 tbsp coconut oil
- 1 tbsp maple syrup
- 1 tsp cinnamon
- ½ tsp sea salt

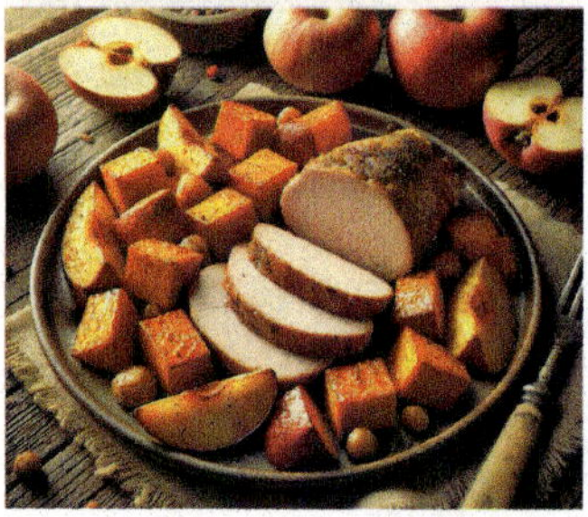

DIRECTIONS

1. Preheat oven to 375°F (190°C).
2. Rub pork with olive oil and season generously with spice mix on all sides.
3. Drizzle apple and sweet potato with melted coconut oil and maple syrup. Toss with cinnamon and sea salt.
4. Place tenderloin, apple slices, and sweet potato cubeson lined baking sheet. Roast 25-30 minutes.
5. Once pork reaches 145°F, remove from oven and let rest for 5-10 minutes.
6. Slice tenderloin into medallions.

NUTRITION

- Calories: 450
- Macros: 15g fat, 40g carbs, 35g protein

Lean pork, paired with caramelized apples and sweet potatoes, creates a nourishing and satisfying dinner.

Lentil and Vegetable Stew with Kale

INGREDIENTS

- 1 tbsp olive oil
- 1 small onion, diced
- 2 cloves garlic
- 1 cup carrots, diced
- 1 cup diced tomatoes
- 1 cup lentils, rinsed
- 4 cups vegetable broth
- 2 cups kale, chopped
- Salt and pepper
- 1 tsp fresh rosemary (or ½ tsp dried)

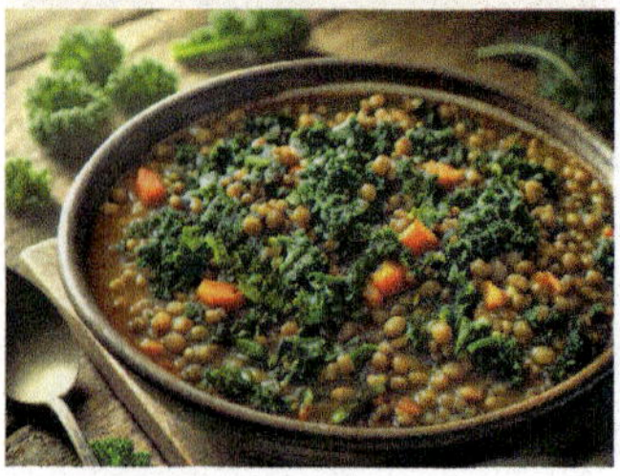

DIRECTIONS

1. In a large pot, sauté onion in olive oil until translucent.
2. Add minced garlic and sauté 1 minute.
3. Add carrots, diced tomatoes, lentils, and broth.
4. Season with salt, pepper, and herbs.
5. Bring to a boil, reduce heat, and simmer for 30-35 minutes or until lentils are tender.
6. Stir in kale and cook for an additional 5 minutes.

NUTRITION

- Calories: 380
- Macros: 10g fat, 55g carbs, 18g protein

This hearty lentil stew is packed with anti-inflammatory ingredients and is perfect for a cozy dinner.

Baked Halibut with Broccoli and Lemon-Garlic Sauce

DIRECTIONS

1. Preheat oven to 400°F (200°C).
2. Drizzle fillets with 1 tbsp olive oil, salt and pepper.
3. Mix 1 tbsp olive oil, garlic, and lemon juice. Pour over halibut fillets.
4. Bake 12-15 minutes, or until opaque and flakes easily with a fork.
5. Steam broccoli in a steamer basket for 5-7 minutes, until bright green and tender-crisp. Add a pinch of salt.
6. Drizzle remaining sauce from baking dish over the fish before serving.
7. Garnish with parsley and lemon slices.

INGREDIENTS

- 2 halibut fillets (6 oz)
- 1 cup broccoli florets
- 2 tbsp olive oil
- Salt and pepper
- 2 cloves of garlic, minced
- Juice of ½ lemon
- Fresh Parsley
- Lemon slices

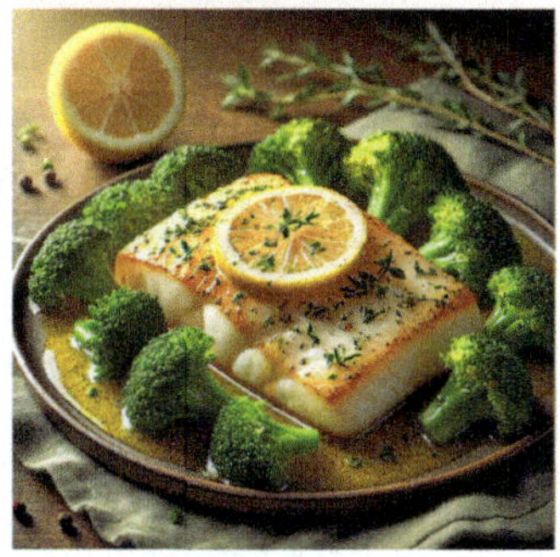

NUTRITION

- Calories: 450
- Macros: 24g fat, 10g carbs, 35g protein

This dish pairs beautifully with a side of brown rice or quinoa.

Lemon-Tahini Chicken with Roasted Veggies

DIRECTIONS

1. Preheat oven to 400°F (200°C).
2. Mix tahini, lemon juice, garlic, salt, and pepper and marinate chicken in mixture for 10-15 minutes.
3. Toss Brussels sprouts and sweet potato with olive oil, salt, and pepper.
4. Spread on baking sheet and roast 25-30 minutes, turning halfway through.
5. Grill marinated chicken breast on oiled grill or grill pan for 6-7 minutes per side, or until cooked through.
6. Garnish with sesame seeds and lemon.

INGREDIENTS

- 2 chicken breasts
- 1 tbsp tahini
- Juice of ½ lemon
- 1 clove garlic, minced
- Salt and pepper
- 1 cup Brussels sprouts, halved
- 1 small sweet potato, peeled and cubed
- 1 tbsp olive oil
- Sesame seeds
- Lemon wedges

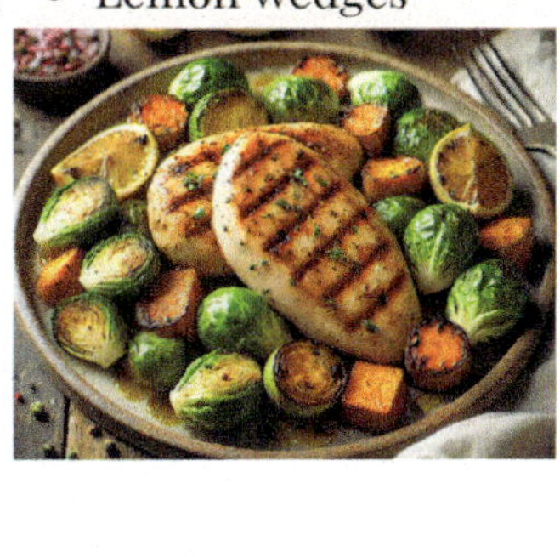

NUTRITION

- Calories: 500
- Macros: 20g fat, 40g carbs, 30g protein

This Mediterranean-inspired dish is both balanced and anti-inflammatory.

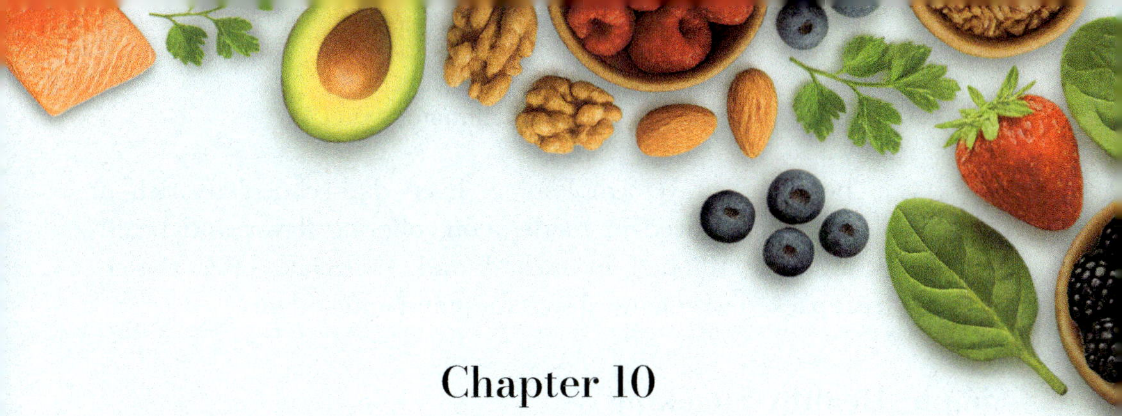

Chapter 10

Anti-Inflammatory Treats and Snacks

In the simplicity of a well-chosen snack or the mindful indulgence in a dessert, we find a subtle yet powerful extension of the anti-inflammatory diet's principles, a reinforcement of our commitment to wellness that resonates with clarity and purpose.

Anti-inflammatory snacking goes beyond satisfying hunger—it can actively support your body's defense against inflammation. Snacks can bridge nutritional gaps, offering quick, nutrient-dense bites that complement your meals.

Indulgence Without Guilt

Sweet treats can still have a place in an anti-inflammatory lifestyle when chosen wisely. Desserts can become nourishing and indulgent when you shift your focus to natural ingredients like fruits and healthy fats. A fruit smoothie can serve as a refreshing snack and satisfy your sweet tooth. A parfait layered with berries and chia pudding provides antioxidants and healthy fats.

Snacks can be decadent yet wholesome. Even dark chocolate, rich in polyphenols, can be enjoyed in moderation, offering flavor and health benefits. Strawberries dipped in melted dark chocolate offer a rich, satisfying treat packed with natural sweetness and antioxidants.

Simple, Healthy Snacking

Adding dips, spreads, and simple, nutrient-dense snacks to your routine can make snacking enjoyable and beneficial for managing inflammation. Options like creamy tzatziki or roasted red pepper and walnut dip provide satisfying flavors and pair well with vegetables or whole-grain crackers for a nutritious, anti-inflammatory boost. Try pairing apple slices with almond butter for a quick and balanced snack, combining fiber and healthy fats that provide energy and calm inflammation.

Whole foods also play a significant role in healthy snacking. Bell pepper slices with homemade hummus, a handful of nuts or seeds, and roasted chickpeas seasoned with olive oil, garlic, and paprika are all flavorful, anti-inflammatory snacks. These options are easy to prepare and offer a range of nutrients that support the body's defenses.

To make snacking easier on busy days, consider prepping ahead with energy balls made from dates, oats, flaxseeds, and almond butter, or homemade granola bars packed with oats, almonds, pumpkin seeds, and dried fruits. These options keep you fueled throughout the day and adhere to anti-inflammatory principles.

Hydration is equally important for an anti-inflammatory lifestyle. Adding cucumber, lemon, or mint to water creates a refreshing drink that not only supports hydration but also helps to reduce inflammation naturally. Simple choices like these make it easier to incorporate anti-inflammatory foods and habits into daily life, keeping snacks healthy, satisfying, and in line with wellness goals.

Anti-inflammatory Treats and Snacks - Recipes

When choosing anti-inflammatory snacks and treats, indulgence and health can go hand-in-hand. Each option, whether a quick snack or a carefully prepared one, becomes an opportunity to nourish your body and support its natural fight against inflammation.

A schedule of snack options follows, with calories and macronutrients listed according to portion size. Recipes for the more complex snacks follow. As always, adjust the suggested snacks and treats to your liking and food tolerances. Enjoy and healthy snacking!

Daily Snacks - Week 1

Day	Snack	Cal	Fat	Carb	Pro
Day 1	1 medium apple, sliced 1 tbsp almond butter	180	9g	25g	3g
	1 medium carrot, cut into sticks 2 celery stalks, cut into sticks ¼ cup hummus	150	8g	15g	4g
Day 2	¼ cup mixed nuts (almonds, walnuts, cashews)	200	18g	9g	6g
	1 cucumber, sliced ¼ cup guacamole	130	10g	12g	2g
Day 3	1 bell pepper, sliced ¼ cup tzatziki (chapter 6)	100	6g	10g	3g
	1 cup fresh pineapple chunks	180	0g	20g	1g
Day 4	1 pear, sliced ¼ cup walnuts	200	15g	24g	3g
	1 cup mixed berries (strawberries, blueberries, raspberries)	60	0g	15g	1g
Day 5	1 orange, peeled and sliced ¼ cup almonds	200	10g	26g	6g
	1 cup sliced radishes and cucumbers ¼ cup hummus (chapter 6)	100	6g	10g	3g
Day 6	Smoothie (blend all ingredients): 1 cup spinach ½ cup frozen mango ½ cup frozen pineapple 1 tbsp chia seeds 1 cup coconut water	220	4g	50g	4g
	1 cup sliced bell peppers ½ cup cherry tomatoes	50	0g	12g	2g
Day 7	1 cup watermelon slices (if in season) 1 tbsp pumpkin seeds	80	2g	18g	2g
	1 square dark chocolate (70% cocoa) 1 cup green tea	60	4g	5g	1g

Daily Snacks - Week 2

Day	Snack	Cal	Fat	Carb	Pro
Day 8	1 pear, sliced ¼ cup walnuts ¼ tsp cinnamon	200	14g	27g	3g
	½ cup roasted chickpeas (see recipe)	150	8g	15g	5g
Day 9	1 bell pepper, sliced ¼ cup guacamole (chapter 6)	150	11g	16g	2g
	1 cup fresh pineapple chunks 1 tbsp unsweetened coconut flakes	90	2g	23g	1g
Day 10	1 cucumber, sliced 2 carrots, sliced into sticks 2 tbsp tahini dip (chapter 6)	150	10g	15g	3g
	1 cup mango slices 1 tsp chia seeds ½ lime, juiced	100	1g	26g	1g
Day 11	¼ cup Brazil nuts 2 tbsp dark chocolate chips	200	16g	16g	4g
	1 cup blueberries ½ cup coconut yogurt	120	4g	20g	2g
Day 12	1 apple, sliced 1 tbsp pumpkin seeds ¼ tsp cinnamon	150	5g	29g	2g
	1 hard-boiled egg ½ cup cherry tomatoes	90	6g	5g	7g
Day 13	1 orange, sliced ¼ cup almonds	180	10g	24g	6g
	Homemade Granola Bar (see recipe)	180	9g	23g	4g
Day 14	1 cup strawberries 2 squares dark chocolate, melted	180	7g	18g	2g
	2 celery stalks, cut into sticks 2 tbsp natural peanut butter 1 tbsp raisins	180	12g	18g	5g

Daily Snacks - Week 3

Day	Snack	Cal	Fat	Carb	Pro
Day 15	1 grapefruit, segmented 1 tsp honey Fresh mint leaves, chopped	90	0g	23g	1g
	1 cup Baked Sweet Potato Chips (see recipe)	150	5g	26g	2g
Day 16	1 cucumber, sliced 2 tbsp olive tapenade	100	7g	8g	2g
	2 celery stalks, cut into sticks 2 tbsp cashew butter 2 dates, chopped	180	10g	20g	4g
Day 17	3 fresh apricots, halved ¼ cup almonds	150	8g	20g	4g
	½ cup low-fat cottage cheese ¼ cup fresh pineapple chunks	110	3g	13g	10g
Day 18	1 apple, sliced 1 tbsp almond butter 1 tbsp hemp seeds	180	9g	25g	4g
	1 cup cantaloupe, sliced Juice of ½ lime	60	0g	15g	1g
Day 19	¼ cup pumpkin seeds	90	7g	4g	5g
	1 cup raspberries 2 tbsp dark chocolate chips	100	4g	20g	2g
Day 20	4 fresh figs, halved 2 tbsp goat cheese	150	6g	24g	4g
	1 cup radishes, sliced ¼ cup guacamole (Chapter 6)	120	8g	12g	2g
Day 21	1 cup blackberries ½ cup Greek yogurt	130	4g	20g	6g
	¼ cup sunflower seeds 2 tbsp dried cranberries	150	7g	20g	5g

Daily Snacks - Week 4

Day	Snack	Cal	Fat	Carb	Pro
Day 22	1 pear, sliced ¼ cup ricotta cheese 2 tbsp walnuts, chopped	180	8g	24g	6g
	1 slice whole-grain bread ½ avocado, mashed Pinch of sea salt and pepper	180	12g	18g	3g
Day 23	¼ cup beet hummus (chapter 6) 1 cucumber, sliced	180	8g	24g	6g
	1 cup fresh pineapple, diced ½ tsp chili powder	80	0g	21g	1g
Day 24	1 cup papaya, diced Juice of 1 lime 1 tbsp unsweetened coconut flakes	90	2g	23g	1g
	1 cup cherry tomatoes, halved 1 tbsp balsamic glaze 2 tbsp fresh basil, chopped	70	3g	14g	1g
Day 25	1 bell pepper, sliced ¼ cup guacamole (chapter 6)	120	8g	12g	2g
	1 cup watermelon, diced 1 tbsp fresh mint, chopped	60	0g	15g	1g
Day 26	1 kiwi, sliced 1 tbsp hemp seeds	70	3g	15g	2g
	1 homemade energy ball (see recipe)	100	6g	12g	2g
Day 27	1 apple, sliced 1 tbsp almond butter	190	9g	28g	3g
	1 cup raspberries ¼ cup almonds	130	8g	18g	4g
Day 28	4 fresh figs, halved 2 tbsp almond butter	180	9g	28g	4g
	2 squares dark chocolate 4 Brazil nuts	180	14g	12g	3g

Roasted Spiced Chickpeas

INGREDIENTS

- 1 cup chickpeas
- 1 tbsp olive oil
- ½ tsp garlic powder
- ½ tsp paprika
- Salt to taste

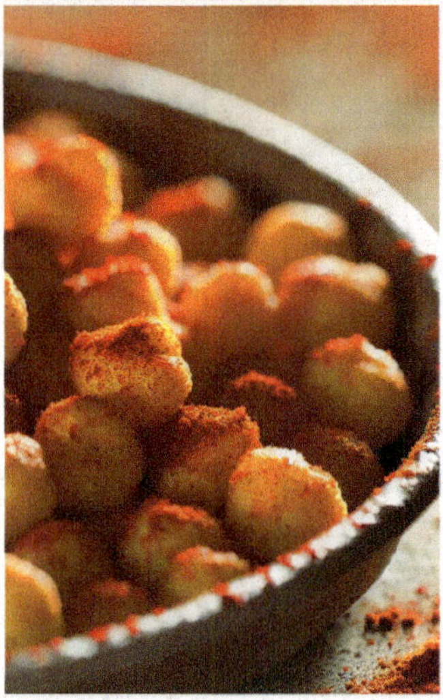

DIRECTIONS

1. Preheat oven to 400°F (200°C).
2. Drain and rinse chickpeas, then pat dry with a paper towel .
3. Toss the chickpeas with olive oil, garlic powder, paprika, and salt until evenly coated.
4. Spread chickpeas over lined baking sheet.
5. Roast for 20-25 minutes, stirring halfway through, until chickpeas are golden and crispy.
6. Allow to cool slightly before serving. They will become crispier as they cool.

NUTRITION

- Calories: 150 (for ½ batch)
- Macros: 8g fat, 15g carbs, 5g protein

This crunchy, flavorful snack is packed with fiber and protein. Try them as a salad topper.

Baked Sweet Potato Chips

INGREDIENTS

- 1 medium sweet potato, thinly sliced
- 1 tbsp olive oil
- Salt to taste

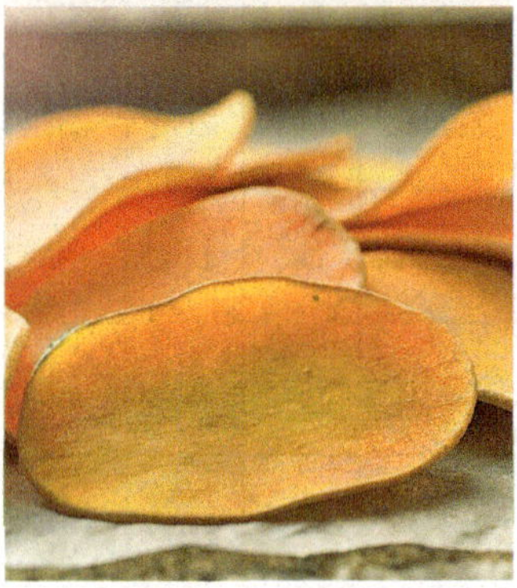

DIRECTIONS

1. Preheat oven to 375°F (190°C).
2. Toss sweet potato slices with olive oil.
3. Sprinkle with salt.
4. Bake for 15-20 minutes until crispy.

NUTRITION

- Calories: 150
- Macros: 5g fat, 26g carbs, 2g protein

These crispy, baked chips are a satisfying snack alternative to other fried options.

Homemade Granola Bars with Oats, Almonds, Pumpkin Seeds, and Dried Fruits

DIRECTIONS

1. Preheatoven to 350°F (175°C).
2. Combine oats, chopped almonds, and pumpkin seeds on a lined baking sheet and toast for 8-10 minutes, stirring halfway through.
3. Warm almond butter, honey, vanilla, cinnamon, and salt in small saucepan. Stir constantly until smooth and well combined.
4. Transfer toasted oat mixture into a large bowl. Add dried fruits and pour almond butter mixture over the top. Stir until well coated.
5. Press the granola mixture firmly and evenly into an 8x8 inch baking dish lined with parcgment paper (leave an overhang for easy removal).
6. Refrigerate for at least 1 hour, or until firm. Once set, lift the bars out of the pan and cut into 12 squares or bars.
7. Store in an airtight container in the refrigerator for up to 1 week, or freeze for longer storage.

INGREDIENTS

- 2 cups rolled oats
- ½ cup raw almonds, chopped
- ¼ cup pumpkin seeds
- ¼ cup dried cranberries or raisins (unsweetened)
- ¼ cup dried apricots, chopped
- ⅓ cup almond butter (or nut butter of choice)
- ¼ cup honey or maple syrup
- 1 tsp vanilla extract
- ¼ tsp cinnamon
- Pinch of salt

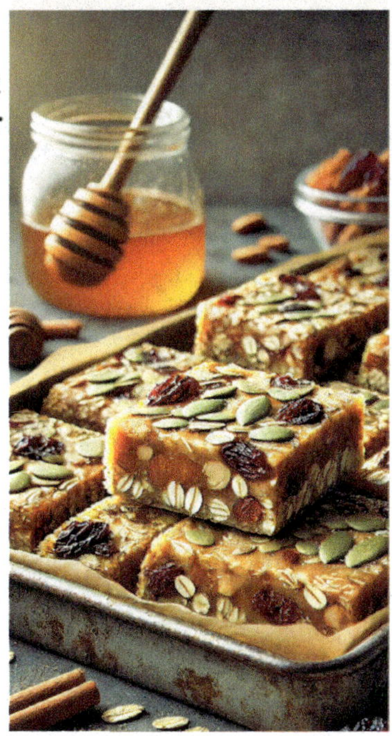

NUTRITION

- Calories (per 1 bar of12): 180
- Macros: 9g fat, 23g carbs, 4g protein

These granola bars are a healthy, anti-inflammatory snack, perfect for a quick energy boost or treat.

Energy Balls with Dates, Oats, Flaxseeds, and Almond Butter

INGREDIENTS

- 1 cup Medjool dates, pitted
- ½ cup rolled oats
- ¼ cup ground flaxseeds
- ¼ cup almond butter
- 1 tsp vanilla extract
- 1 tbsp chia seeds (optional, for extra texture and nutrients)
- 2 tbsp dark chocolate chips (optional)
- Pinch of salt

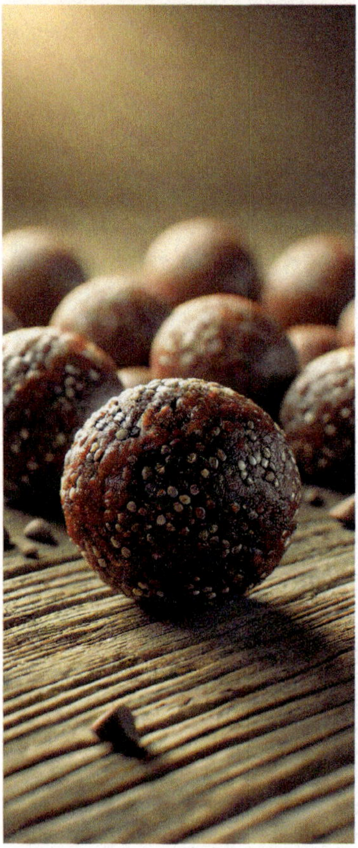

DIRECTIONS

1. If the dates are a bit dry, soak them in warm water for 10 minutes to soften. Drain well.
2. In a food processor, combine the pitted dates, rolled oats, ground flaxseeds, almond butter, vanilla extract, and a pinch of salt.
3. Pulse until the mixture becomes a sticky, dough-like consistency. If adding chia seeds or dark chocolate chips, fold them into the mixture by hand.
4. Scoop out about 1 tablespoon of the mixture and roll it between your palms to form a ball. Repeat with the remaining mixture.
5. Place the energy balls on a parchment-lined baking sheet or plate and refrigerate for about 20-30 minutes to firm up.
6. Once set, transfer the energy balls to an airtight container.
7. They can be stored in the fridge for up to 1 week or frozen for longer storage.

NUTRITION

- Calories (per 1 inch ball): 100
- Macros: 6g fat, 12g carbs, 2g protein

These energy balls are a convenient and nutritious snack option, perfect for pre- or post-workout fuel or as a quick energy boost during busy days!

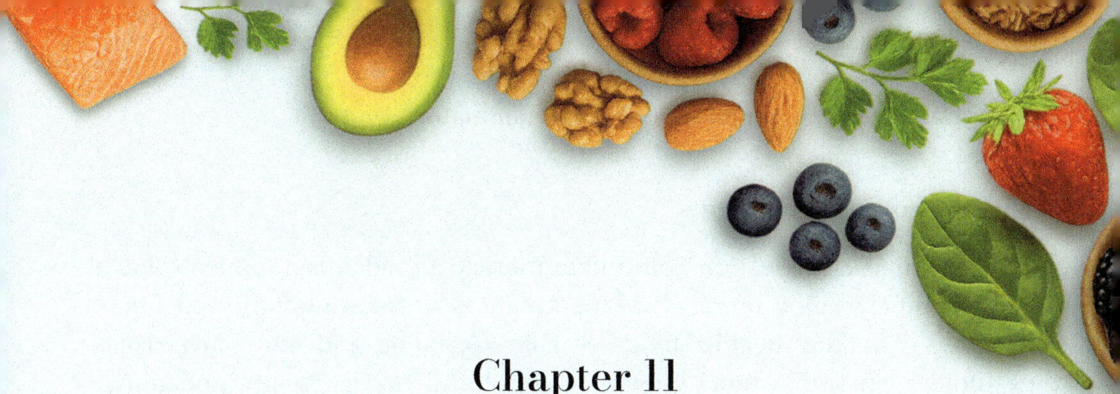

Chapter 11

Tailoring the Anti-Inflammatory Diet for Every Table

Every table tells its own story, rich with the traditions, tastes, and textures that define those who gather around it. With thoughtful adjustments and personal touches, this way of eating becomes more than a list of ingredients—it transforms into a flexible, nourishing ritual that respects individual choices, no matter who has gathered around the table.

In the flow of daily routines, meal planning often becomes the task of a single family member. Yet, when everyone participates, it becomes an opportunity to connect and create together. Picture a Saturday morning at the market, where each family member is invited to pick out one anti-inflammatory ingredient they enjoy. With each person contributing their own choice to the week's meals, grocery shopping becomes an engaging experience. It's a fun way to learn about healthy eating, and it makes every meal feel like a shared success, as each ingredient represents the input of the whole family.

Kid-Approved Recipes

Transforming nutrient-rich, anti-inflammatory ingredients into meals that kids genuinely enjoy requires a balance of taste, presentation, and fun. The key is making healthy foods visually appealing and interactive. For example, a smoothie bowl topped with colorful berries, seeds, and nuts becomes a canvas for kids to create their own designs, turning breakfast into an artful, hands-on activity. Another favorite is "zoodle" spaghetti—spiralized zucchini noodles served with homemade marinara sauce—which brings a playful twist to pasta night while sneaking in extra veggies.

Involving kids in meal prep is also a powerful way to spark curiosity and encourage healthy choices. Teaching them about why certain foods are good for their bodies, like explaining the benefits of omega-3s as you prepare baked salmon or discussing the nutrients in colorful veggies while making a rainbow veggie pizza, makes nutrition accessible and relatable. When kids understand the "why" behind healthy choices, it fosters a natural interest. It sets the stage for lifelong healthy eating habits. This hands-on, approachable method helps kids see nutritious food not as a requirement but as an exciting part of their everyday lives.

Balancing Different Preferences, Needs, and Cultural Backgrounds

Tailoring the anti-inflammatory diet to fit the preferences, needs, and cultural backgrounds of everyone at the table allows this approach to become more inclusive and sustainable. Rather than following rigid guidelines, customizing meals to reflect family traditions and dietary requirements adds depth and meaning to an anti-inflammatory lifestyle. This flexibility helps create a way of eating that's health-supportive, relevant, and enjoyable for each person, regardless of age or background.

A key strategy in tailoring the anti-inflammatory diet is to incorporate flavors, ingredients, and dishes that resonate with family traditions and personal tastes. For example, if spicy foods are popular in the household, anti-inflammatory spices like turmeric, ginger, and cayenne pepper can be incorporated into dishes, enhancing flavor while providing health benefits.

Incorporating olive oil, fresh herbs, garlic, and roasted vegetables for families who enjoy Mediterranean flavors can make meals feel familiar yet remain anti-inflammatory. Adjusting recipes to align with personal or cultural preferences helps the diet feel like an extension of one's identity rather than a restrictive change.

Including a variety of proteins and plant-based options also allows the anti-inflammatory diet to be more versatile and accessible. Providing a range of protein sources is essential in homes where different dietary practices exist—like vegetarian, pescatarian, or omnivorous diets. Legumes, tofu, fatty fish, and lean meats can each serve as a base for different dishes, offering variety and balance. These options allow each family member to incorporate anti-inflammatory foods into their diet while honoring their unique dietary needs.

One way to make the anti-inflammatory diet adaptable for every table is to approach meal preparation as a modular process. Preparing several ingredients—such as roasted vegetables, grains, greens, and proteins—allows for easy mix-and-match meals that can be assembled differently for each person. A base of greens or grains can be topped with various proteins and dressings, offering flexibility while reducing prep time. This setup also encourages each family member to build a plate that meets their specific preferences, fostering a sense of autonomy and satisfaction.

Tailoring the anti-inflammatory diet involves experimenting with food pairings and cooking techniques that bring out the best in nutrient-dense ingredients. Roasting, grilling, or steaming vegetables can enhance their natural flavors, making them more appealing, especially for picky eaters. Trying new combinations, like serving berries with yogurt and nuts for breakfast or making a colorful veggie stir-fry, invites variety and enjoyment. Making the anti-inflammatory diet flexible and flavorful becomes a way of eating that supports everyone's health and enjoyment, turning each meal into an opportunity to nourish both body and spirit.

Combining Anti-Inflammatory and Weight Loss Goals

Combining weight loss goals with an anti-inflammatory diet naturally aligns two health priorities to support overall well-being and long-term balance. This approach emphasizes nutrient-dense foods that help regulate inflammation and contribute to feelings of fullness and satisfaction, reducing the need for restrictive calorie counting. Rather than focusing solely on calories, it encourages selecting foods that nourish deeply, offering high nutritional value per bite. This shift away from traditional calorie-focused dieting helps foster a relationship with food that values quality over quantity, making weight loss achievable and sustainable.

At the heart of this combined approach are foods naturally high in vitamins, minerals, antioxidants, and anti-inflammatory compounds. Leafy greens, colorful berries, fatty fish, whole grains, and nuts all play a central role, bringing together essential fiber, healthy fats, and protein to regulate appetite and sustain energy. These foods help maintain stable blood sugar levels, reducing sudden cravings and promoting steady energy throughout the day. By addressing both physical and mental satiety, they encourage mindful choices that align with both weight management and inflammation reduction.

Regular physical activity further supports this approach, adding momentum to weight loss goals while reinforcing the benefits of anti-inflammatory eating. Movement—whether a brisk walk, yoga, or strength training—enhances metabolic health, boosts insulin sensitivity, and encourages fat loss. Exercise also complements the diet by reducing inflammation and fostering a resilient, balanced body. This partnership between nourishing foods and physical activity forms a strong foundation, allowing weight loss to occur naturally while supporting overall vitality.

Mindful eating introduces another dimension to this journey, bringing awareness to the body's hunger and fullness cues. By focusing on internal signals rather than external cues—such as portion sizes or set meal times—mindful eating allows for a more balanced approach to food. Each meal becomes an opportunity to slow down, savor flavors, and register fullness, naturally reducing the likelihood of overeating. This practice encourages a mindful relationship with food that values quality over speed, reinforcing both satiety and satisfaction.

By combining the principles of anti-inflammatory eating with weight loss goals, we move beyond the idea of restriction and embrace a model of nourishment and balance. This holistic approach acknowledges the interconnectedness of the body's systems, from gut health to hormone regulation. It aligns dietary choices with the body's natural rhythms for healing and renewal. The result is a path toward weight management that is sustainable and enriched by a deeper understanding of food's role in promoting health. In choosing nutrient-dense foods, engaging in regular movement, and practicing mindful eating, this approach offers a comprehensive, fulfilling, and health-focused way to achieve weight goals while honoring the body's need for balance and wellness.

Managing Autoimmune Conditions with Diet

The connection between diet and the management of autoimmune conditions lies in the body's complex systems, where what we eat can either ease or worsen autoimmune symptoms. Central to this interaction is the gut—a hub of immune function and nutrient absorption—where the foods we consume can support the gut's protective barrier and foster a balanced microbiome or, conversely, contribute to a weakened barrier and trigger inflammation. The gut's role in autoimmune health makes dietary choices particularly impactful for those with autoimmune conditions.

The Autoimmune Protocol (AIP) diet offers a targeted approach to help manage autoimmune conditions. This protocol is stricter than the general anti-inflammatory diet. It is designed to eliminate common dietary triggers, such as nightshades, nuts, seeds, and eggs, in addition to processed foods and added sugars. By focusing on nutrient-dense foods, the AIP diet aims to heal the gut, regulate immune responses, and reduce symptoms associated with autoimmune flare-ups. For those with autoimmune challenges, the AIP diet represents a structured path toward relief by addressing the root triggers of inflammation.

Personalizing the AIP diet is essential, as each person's response to food can vary significantly. The diet begins with a strict elimination phase, followed by a gradual reintroduction of foods, allowing individuals to identify specific triggers that may exacerbate their symptoms. This reintroduction phase requires patience and careful observation, as each food is added back into the diet one at a time, with its effects on the body closely monitored. This process enables individuals to build a sustainable, long-term eating plan that minimizes autoimmune symptoms without unnecessary restrictions, creating a diet tailored to their unique needs.

Given the intricacies of autoimmune diseases, working with a healthcare provider is often necessary. These professionals provide guidance, helping ensure the diet is safe and nutritionally balanced. They also assist in tracking symptoms and making dietary adjustments as needed, offering insights that might be difficult to identify alone. This collaboration becomes especially valuable for managing potential nutrient deficiencies and understanding symptom patterns, particularly when symptoms overlap with other conditions.

For individuals following the AIP diet, active engagement with their health becomes essential. Tracking symptoms through food and symptom diaries can reveal connections between certain foods and symptom flare-ups, highlighting patterns that empower individuals to make informed dietary choices. This self-awareness, combined with professional guidance, helps those with autoimmune conditions actively participate in their own care.

As people follow the AIP diet, its effects on managing autoimmune symptoms can be gradual, sometimes subtle, but meaningful. While the AIP diet does not claim to cure autoimmune diseases, it offers a practical strategy for reducing symptoms and improving quality of life. The diet underscores the therapeutic potential of food, showing that dietary choices can be a valuable part of a comprehensive approach to managing autoimmune conditions. By embracing the principles of the AIP diet, individuals with autoimmune diseases can find a path to wellness that complements medical treatments, making food an ally in the pursuit of a balanced and resilient life.

The Role of Anti-Inflammatory Eating in Athletic Success

Athletes push their bodies to the limit, requiring energy, quick recovery, and lasting resilience. An anti-inflammatory diet can play a significant role in helping them perform at their best, supporting energy, managing inflammation, and aiding recovery after intense workouts. By focusing on balanced nutrition, timing meals around training, and staying hydrated, athletes can give their bodies the support they need for peak performance.

For athletes, proteins, carbohydrates, and fats each have specific jobs. Protein is essential for muscle repair and growth, so getting enough daily protein helps muscles recover and stay strong. Carbohydrates are the primary source of energy for high-intensity activities. They are vital for refueling the body after workouts, especially when choosing complex carbs like whole grains, which release energy steadily. Fats are also important for long-lasting energy and fighting inflammation, with foods rich in omega-3s—like salmon, flaxseeds, and walnuts being particularly helpful.

Another critical factor is meal timing. Eating a balanced meal or snack, including carbohydrates and protein, before a workout helps fuel the body and prevent fatigue. After training, there's a "golden hour" when the body is primed for recovery, making this the best time to eat a meal with protein to repair muscles and carbohydrates to replenish energy stores. This timing helps ensure the body has what it needs to recover and prepare for the next workout.

Anti-inflammatory foods are especially helpful during recovery. After intense exercise, the body needs to repair muscles and reduce inflammation. Foods like tart cherries and turmeric have compounds that help reduce soreness and inflammation, and omega-3 supplements from fish oil or algae provide a concentrated dose of anti-inflammatory fats that can support recovery.

Staying hydrated is crucial, too. Proper hydration helps muscles work efficiently, supports heart health, and keeps the mind sharp during exercise. Replacing electrolytes lost through sweat with drinks like coconut water or low-sugar electrolyte drinks helps maintain hydration, especially in hot conditions or during long workouts.

Finally, managing energy through smart eating is essential for athletes. A light, balanced pre-workout meal, like a piece of whole-grain toast with almond butter, provides steady energy. For long workouts, snacks like a banana or an energy bar can help keep energy levels up. After exercise, a meal with protein and carbs—like a smoothie with Greek yogurt and berries—supports muscle recovery and replenishes energy.

This approach to nutrition is intended to support every part of an athlete's training routine, helping them stay strong, recover well, and keep their energy levels steady. With an anti-inflammatory diet, athletes can feel more resilient and perform at their best, giving their bodies the support they need for both short-term goals and long-term wellness.

A Celebration of Wellness and Community

Tailoring the anti-inflammatory diet for every table is about more than just choosing specific foods—it's a commitment to a lifestyle that prioritizes health, flavor, and mindful eating. Integrating nutrient-rich ingredients, seasonal produce, and balanced meals into our routines creates a foundation that supports our well-being and invites others to join us. This approach isn't restrictive but instead offers a variety of flavors, textures, and nutrients that make each meal an opportunity to nourish the body and enjoy the moment.

By adopting anti-inflammatory principles, we share a table that reflects our values, promotes vitality, and connects us with others. With this diet as our guide, we cultivate a way of eating that benefits our health and brings people together, transforming the simple act of sharing a meal into a celebration of wellness and community.

Share Your Experience

> "As we let our own light shine, we unconsciously give others permission to do the same."
>
> — Marianne Williamson

As we near the conclusion of *Calm Your Inflammation Anti-inflammatory Diet,* I hope the recipes, strategies, and guidance shared within these pages have brought you closer to a healthier, more vibrant life. If you've found value in this book—whether it's a recipe that became a favorite, a tip that made a difference, or a new understanding of anti-inflammatory living—I'd love to hear about it.

Your story is important and has the power to inspire others on their journey to health. By leaving a review on Amazon.com, you can share your experience and help others discover the benefits of calming their inflammation through simple, practical changes.

It only takes a minute to share your thoughts.

You can pop over to Amazon with this link:

https://www.amazon.com/review/review-your-purchases/?asin=1963554035

Or scan this QR code with the camera on your phone and touch the link that pops up. The rest is even easier! Just follow the prompts to leave your review. It takes less than 60 seconds!

Thank you for being part of this journey and for choosing to invest in your health. Together, we can inspire others to take the first step toward a healthier, happier future.

Warmest Regards,
Brenda

Conclusion

Next Steps in Anti-Inflammatory Living

An anti-inflammatory diet is a practical, empowering way to nurture both body and mind, transforming the way you feel daily. When inflammation is kept in check, you're more likely to experience stable energy levels, improved mood, and reduced aches and pains. Unlike many diets that focus on short-term results, anti-inflammatory eating centers around long-term wellness, helping you feel your best not just today but for years to come.

This way of eating isn't just a trend; it's a proactive approach to long-term health that addresses the root causes of many chronic conditions. By focusing on nutrient-dense, whole foods, this lifestyle helps reduce systemic inflammation that can lead to issues like heart disease, diabetes, and arthritis. Prioritizing foods rich in antioxidants, healthy fats, and fiber strengthens your immune system and creates a foundation for sustained well-being. It's a small yet impactful change that accumulates over time, enhancing the quality of life through improved energy, mental clarity, and physical resilience.

This approach also brings a positive shift in your relationship with food. Moving away from heavily processed foods toward fresh, wholesome ingredients invites a renewed appreciation for cooking and eating. The vibrant flavors, textures, and aromas of anti-inflammatory foods enhance the joy of mealtime and make nourishing your body a satisfying experience. This mindful connection with food promotes balance and moderation, where enjoying meals isn't about restriction but about embracing a way of eating that supports your health.

An anti-inflammatory lifestyle encourages continuous learning and adaptability as nutrition science evolves and new insights emerge. Staying open to exploring different foods, cooking methods, and meal-planning strategies keeps your approach fresh and engaging. This adaptability fosters a sustainable and enjoyable lifestyle, where anti-inflammatory eating becomes second nature, blending seamlessly into everyday life. Embracing this lifestyle is a commitment to lifelong wellness, grounded in small, meaningful choices that enhance both personal health and a sense of connection to the broader world.

Fortunately, there are many resources available, from scientific journals to online courses focused on nutrition and wellness. Each article you read, and class you attend deepens your understanding and strengthens your commitment to anti-inflammatory living. Over time, you'll build your own knowledge and share what you learn with others, becoming a source of support and information within your community.

Connecting with others committed to an anti-inflammatory lifestyle can provide invaluable support and ideas. From local health food co-ops and cooking classes to online forums, these communities offer spaces to share experiences, recipes, and strategies that work. By participating, you enrich your knowledge and contribute to a broader knowledge pool that makes this lifestyle accessible to others.

Advocacy and education can become natural parts of this commitment. Sharing your experiences through conversations, local events, and social media helps raise awareness and inspires others to explore anti-inflammatory living. By discussing both the science behind these practices and the personal benefits, you can encourage positive changes for individual health, the community, and the environment.

This book has explored a range of tools for anti-inflammatory living, from meal planning and culinary techniques to lifelong learning and community engagement. As you move forward, remember that this isn't a rigid set of rules but a flexible path for growth, discovery, and sharing. Reflecting on this process often reveals a more profound impact on your life, from better health and energy to a greater sense of connection with food and the natural world. This reflection highlights the value of your commitment and reinforces the motivation to continue.

Finally, adopting an anti-inflammatory way of eating empowers you to take control of your health in a meaningful way. Each meal becomes an opportunity to support your body and reinforce positive habits. Rather than restrictive or complicated, this approach offers flexibility and variety, allowing you to enjoy a rich range of flavors while prioritizing foods that promote healing. Embracing anti-inflammatory eating isn't about perfection; it's about consistently making choices that serve your health, your goals, and the world around you.

Bibliography

American Autoimmune Related Diseases Association. (n.d.). *Culinary medicine: Autoimmunity and healthful eating*. Retrieved from https://www.autoimmuneinstitute.org/articles/living-well/culinary-medicine-autoimmunity-and-healthful-eating/

Bach, A., & Ginsburg, S. (2020). *Chronic inflammation in the context of everyday life*. National Center for Biotechnology Information. Retrieved from https://www.ncbi.nlm.nih.-gov/pmc/articles/PMC7312944/

Consumer Reports. (n.d.). *Anti-inflammatory foods from around the world*. Retrieved from https://www.consumerreports.org/health/anti-inflammatory-foods-from-around-the-world-a5899420098/

Dr. Greg Wells. (2023, May 22). 6 ways to decrease stress-induced inflammation. *DrGregWells.com*. Retrieved from https://drgregwells.com/blog/6-ways-to-decrease-stress-induced-inflammation

DrWeil.com. (n.d.). *Dr. Weil's anti-inflammatory diet*. Retrieved from https://www.dr-weil.com/diet-nutrition/anti-inflammatory-diet-pyramid/dr-weils-anti-inflammatory-diet/

EatingWell. (2023, May 22). *15+ dietitian-approved budget-friendly anti-inflammatory meals*. Retrieved from https://www.eatingwell.com/gallery/7965257/dietitian-budget-anti-inflammatory-recipes/

EatingWell. (2023, May 22). *25 anti-inflammatory breakfasts in 15 minutes*. Retrieved from https://www.eatingwell.com/gallery/7916792/anti-inflammatory-breakfasts-in-15-minutes/

EatingWell. (2023, May 22). *30-day anti-inflammatory diet meal plan*. Retrieved from https://www.eatingwell.com/article/7866186/30-day-anti-inflammatory-meal-plan/

EatingWell. (2023, May 22). *38 anti-inflammatory dinners you can make in 30 minutes*. Retrieved from https://www.eatingwell.com/gallery/7946056/anti-inflammatory-dinner-recipes-in-30-minutes/

EatingWell. (2023, May 22). *The 6 best budget-friendly anti-inflammatory foods*. Retrieved from https://www.eatingwell.com/article/8024844/best-budget-friendly-anti-inflammatory-foods/

Gut Microbiota for Health. (n.d.). *Probiotics and anti-inflammatory effects in chronic intestinal diseases*. Retrieved from https://www.gutmicrobiotaforhealth.com/can-probiotics-have-anti-inflammatory-effects-worth-considering-in-chronic-intestinal-diseases/

Harvard Health Publishing. (2021, November 30). *Anti-inflammatory food superstars for every season*. Retrieved from https://www.health.harvard.edu/blog/anti-inflammatory-food-superstars-for-every-season-202111302648

Harvard T.H. Chan School of Public Health. (n.d.). *Diet review: Anti-inflammatory diet*. The Nutrition Source. Retrieved from https://www.hsph.harvard.edu/nutrition-source/healthy-weight/diet-reviews/anti-inflammatory-diet/

Harvard T.H. Chan School of Public Health. (n.d.). *Mindful eating*. The Nutrition Source. Retrieved from https://www.hsph.harvard.edu/nutritionsource/mindful-eating/

Healthline. (n.d.). *AIP (Autoimmune Protocol) diet: A beginner's guide.* Retrieved from https://www.healthline.com/nutrition/aip-diet-autoimmune-protocol-diet

Janssen, I. A., & Ross, R. (2010). *Water, hydration, and health.* National Center for Biotechnology Information. Retrieved from https://www.ncbi.nlm.nih.gov/pmc/articles/PMC2908954/

Johns Hopkins Medicine. (n.d.). *Anti-inflammatory diet.* Retrieved from https://www.hopkinsmedicine.org/health/wellness-and-prevention/anti-inflammatory-diet

Krich, J. (2023, May 22). 6 ways to decrease stress-induced inflammation. *Dr. Greg Wells.* Retrieved from https://drgregwells.com/blog/6-ways-to-decrease-stress-induced-inflammation

McKay, D. L., & Blumberg, J. B. (2012). *Omega-3 fatty acids and inflammatory processes.* National Center for Biotechnology Information. Retrieved from https://www.ncbi.nlm.nih.gov/pmc/articles/PMC3257651/

National Center for Biotechnology Information. (2021). *Food allergy and intolerance: A narrative review on pathophysiology, diagnosis, and management.* Retrieved from https://www.ncbi.nlm.nih.gov/pmc/articles/PMC8152468/

National Center for Biotechnology Information. (2022). *Synergistic anti-inflammatory activity of ginger and turmeric.* Retrieved from https://www.ncbi.nlm.nih.gov/pmc/articles/PMC9229778/

Stone, M. J. (2017). Regulation of Chemokine–Receptor Interactions and Functions. International Journal of Molecular Sciences. https://doi.org/10.3390/ijms18112415

About the Author

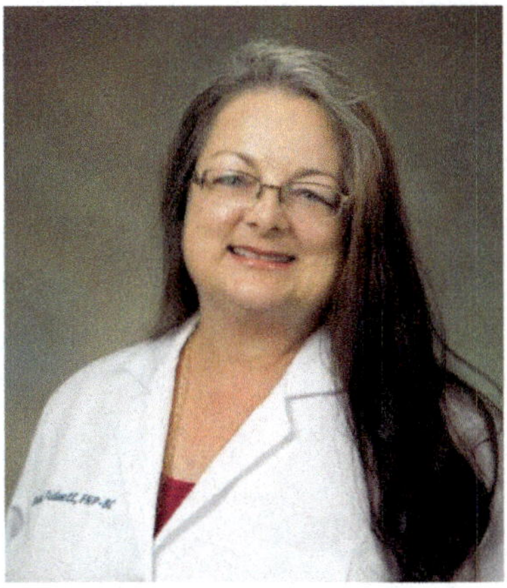

Brenda Tidwell is a devoted wife, mother to two loving sons, and a doting grandmother of four. Her happiest moments are spent surrounded by her family or soaking up the serene natural beauty of the California coast.

In her professional life, Brenda is a seasoned Doctor of Nursing Practice and a board-certified Family Nurse Practitioner with a heart for writing and a focus on wellness. She has a talent for turning complex medical topics into engaging, understandable content that resonates with people from all walks of life. Her books are born from a dedication to helping others understand how lifestyle and dietary choices can combat chronic disease, aiming to enhance overall health.

Her writing is more than just informative—it's a source of empowerment and optimism for those seeking a healthier life. Brenda's unique blend of personal warmth and professional expertise makes her a compelling voice in the conversation about health and well-being.

Also by Dr. Brenda Tidwell

Calm Your Inflammation: 7 Proven Secrets to Regulate Your Immune System, Balance Gut Health, Reduce Stress, and Feel Your Best Every Day

Available on Amazon.com through the QR code below. Just scan this QR code with the camera on your phone and touch the link that pops up.

Calm Your Inflammation 2 Books in 1: Science-Backed Strategies to Enhance Your Immune System, Promote Gut Health, and Feel Your Best Every Day

Available on Amazon.com through the QR code below. Just scan this QR code with the camera on your phone and touch the link that pops up.

Printed in Dunstable, United Kingdom

76939778R00090